WITHDRAWN
USJ Library

Shane P. Desselle, Ph.D.
Dana P. Hammer, Ph.D.
Editors

Handbook for Pharmacy Educators: Getting Adjusted As a New Pharmacy Faculty Member

Handbook for Pharmacy Educators: Getting Adjusted As a New Pharmacy Faculty Member has been co-published simultaneously as *Journal of Pharmacy Teaching*, Volume 9, Number 1 2002.

*Pre-publication
REVIEWS,
COMMENTARIES,
EVALUATIONS...*

"I think that this book would be of value to new faculty in any field, and especially relevant to Pharmacy faculty. The book delves deeply into the battles and worries confronting new faculty, and is written in a conversational style that made me feel that I was talking to the author over a cup of coffee.... I feel that this book would be especially useful for new faculty who, for whatever reason, do not have other new faculty with whom to trade stories. In addition, the book is an excellent treatise on the perceptions of new faculty, and in this way makes excellent reading for chairpersons and higher level administrators who may have forgotten what it was like to get started in academia. I also think the book gives some practical advice on teaching, grading, collegiality, balance, and the pursuit of tenure, that would enlighten graduate students who are considering a career in the 'ivory towers' of academia."

Tom Anchordoquy, Ph.D.
*Assistant Professor
University of Colorado
School of Pharmacy*

More pre-publication
REVIEWS, COMMENTARIES, EVALUATIONS . . .

"The *Handbook for Pharmacy Educators: Getting Adjusted As a New Pharmacy Faculty Member* provides first hand accounts of the first few years in the careers of five new pharmacy academics. With recruitment and retention of pharmacy faculty members being of primary concern for colleges/schools of pharmacy across the country, the topic is a timely one. The five new academics represent diverse academic disciplines and diverse institutions, and therefore, a broad audience of future, new, and mid-career pharmacy educators as well as administrators will benefit from this book. Each chapter provides a personal account of the first few years of the author's career in academia. The accounts are aptly organized around the basic triad of academia: teaching, service, and research/scholarship.

A common theme expressed by each contributor is the importance of mentoring and the need for formal mentoring programs. This piece of information is useful for all readers. The book is a welcome addition to the field of pharmaceutical education."

Michelle M. Kalis, Ph.D.
Associate Dean and
Associate Professor of Pharmacology
School of Pharmacy
Boston, Massachusetts
College of Pharmacy
and Health Sciences

"This book provides many valuable lessons for new faculty members and those aspiring to a career in academe. Furthermore, it offers insight into the challenges faced by any individual who is currently navigating the complexities of an academic career. Therefore, it also has potential application for more experienced members of the academy. A significant strength of the book is that perspectives are offered from several disciplines, institutions, and both genders.

Although each chapter provides useful information and shares experiences from which we all can learn, the chapter authored by Lon Larson stands out is a must read for all faculty, no matter the discipline, academic setting, or level of experience. This chapter serves to remind us of why we do what we do and offers some very sage advice regarding success and fulfillment."

John Bentley, R.Ph., M.B.A., Ph.D.
Assistant Professor
Pharmacy Administration
School of Pharmacy
The University of Mississippi

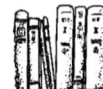

More pre-publication
REVIEWS, COMMENTARIES, EVALUATIONS . . .

"I found the book to be a very introspective account of life as a faculty member that I could relate to on a personal level in many ways and that I could see other colleagues relating to as well. The authors were well-chosen by prominence within the field, breadth and scope of practice. Faculty at all levels will be able to relate to this book on a personal level. This book will serve as a tool for junior faculty to guide them through the first days and months of life on faculty that are often fraught with many unknowns and uncertainty. It will also serve as a guide to laying the foundation for successful promotion, answering many questions before the junior faculty person has to experience them the hard way."

Bradley Tice, Pharm.D.
*Assistant Professor
of Pharmacy Practice
and Director
of the Drake-American Drug Stores
Community Care Laboratory
Drake University*

"*Handbook for Pharmacy Educators: Getting Adjusted As a New Pharmacy Faculty Member*, focuses on a much-needed topic for those entering into a new faculty position. As stated throughout most chapters of the book, most new faculty members enter the academic world with very little experience and knowledge of all that is required for success. A quote very early on from one of the editors sums up what many of us thought when we moved into our first faculty office, 'Well, what do I do, now?' This text provides some very thoughtful answers to this very simple question. . . . I would strongly suggest that this text be read by all new faculty."

Marc W. Harrold, Ph.D.
*Professor of Medicinal Chemistry
Duquesne University
School of Pharmacy
Pittsburgh, Pennsylvania*

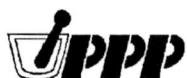

Pharmaceutical Products Press
An Imprint of The Haworth Press, Inc.

Handbook for Pharmacy Educators: Getting Adjusted As a New Pharmacy Faculty Member

Handbook for Pharmacy Educators: Getting Adjusted As a New Pharmacy Faculty Member has been co-published simultaneously as *Journal of Pharmacy Teaching*, Volume 9, Number 1 2002.

The *Journal of Pharmacy Teaching* Monographic "Separates"

Below is a list of "separates," which in serials librarianship means a special issue simultaneously published as a special journal issue or double-issue *and* as a "separate" hardbound monograph. (This is a format which we also call a "DocuSerial.")

"Separates" are published because specialized libraries or professionals may wish to purchase a specific thematic issue by itself in a format which can be separately cataloged and shelved, as opposed to purchasing the journal on an on-going basis. Faculty members may also more easily consider a "separate" for classroom adoption.

"Separates" are carefully classified separately with the major book jobbers so that the journal tie-in can be noted on new book order slips to avoid duplicate purchasing.

You may wish to visit Haworth's website at . . .

http://www.HaworthPress.com

. . . to search our online catalog for complete tables of contents of these separates and related publications.

You may also call 1-800-HAWORTH (outside US/Canada: 607-722-5857), or Fax 1-800-895-0582 (outside US/Canada: 607-771-0012), or e-mail at:

getinfo@haworthpressinc.com

Handbook for Pharmacy Educators: Getting Adjusted As a New Pharmacy Faculty Member, edited by Shane P. Desselle, Ph.D., and Dana P. Hammer, Ph.D. (Vol. 9, No. 1, 2002). *Helps new pharmacy faculty make a smooth transition into academia.*

Handbook for Pharmacy Educators: Contemporary Teaching Principles and Strategies, edited by Noel E. Wilkin, R.Ph., Ph.D. (Vol. 7, No. 3/4, 2000). *The Handbook for Pharmacy Educators will help you develop ways to delineate and assess outcomes projected by the curricula in order to become an effective teacher amidst the changing health care environment. Also for graduate students, this guide offers an abilities-based approach, provides contemporary strategies for facilitating ability acquisition, and describes the process of assessment that will provide feedback regarding the effectiveness of these teaching strategies. Comprehensive and thorough, this book will help you understand the principles of outcome identification and implementation; strategies that will assist you in teaching students the knowledge, skills, and attitudes associated with those outcomes; the principles of assessment-as- learning; and the process of institutionalization of assessment. The Handbook for Pharmacy Educators will help you implement new teaching methods or rethink old ones to successfully face questions and challenges in the dynamic field of pharmacy.*

Teaching and Learning Strategies in Pharmacy Ethics, Second Edition, edited by Amy Marie Haddad, Ph.D. (Vol. 6, No. 1/2, 1997). *"Offers widened access to creative, invigorating scholarship. . . . It is a window into how instruction in the theory and practice of ethical pharmacy practice meets disparate needs in the contemporary academy." (Jonathan J. Wolfe, PhD, Associate Professor of Pharmacy Practice, University of Arkansas for Medical Sciences, Little Rock)*

Ethical Dimensions of Pharmaceutical Care, edited by Amy Marie Haddad, Ph.D., and Robert A. Buerki, Ph.D. (Vol. 5, No. 1/2, 1996). *"Offers a philosophical basis for understanding just what 'care' is, why the profession ought to care about its patients, and different ways of viewing ethical standards in evaluating pharmaceutical care situations. . . . Balances hard, thought-provoking material with situations requiring applied ethics. . . . Aimed at the foundation of pharmacy's future." (American Journal of Pharmaceutical Education)*

Multicultural Pharmaceutical Education, edited by Barry Bleidt, Ph.D. (Vol. 3, No. 2, 1992). *"Provides practical information on programs that have worked in colleges of pharmacy. Useful reading for those who would like to see their pharmacy schools place greater emphasis on multicultural education and for those who question such efforts." (The Annals of Pharmacotherapy)*

Handbook for Pharmacy Educators: Getting Adjusted As a New Pharmacy Faculty Member

Shane P. Desselle, Ph.D.
Dana P. Hammer, Ph.D.
Editors

Handbook for Pharmacy Educators: Getting Adjusted As a New Pharmacy Faculty Member has been co-published simultaneously as *Journal of Pharmacy Teaching*, Volume 9, Number 1 2002.

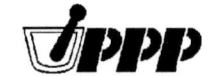

Pharmaceutical Products Press
An Imprint of
The Haworth Press, Inc.
New York • London • Oxford

Published by

The Pharmaceutical Products Press®, 10 Alice Street, Binghamton, NY 13904-1580 USA

The Pharmaceutical Products Press® is an imprint of The Haworth Press, Inc., 10 Alice Street, Binghamton, NY 13904-1580 USA.

Handbook for Pharmacy Educators: Getting Adjusted As a New Pharmacy Faculty Member has been co-published simultaneously as *Journal of Pharmacy Teaching*, Volume 9, Number 1 2002.

©2002 by The Haworth Press, Inc. All rights reserved. No part of this work may be reproduced or utilized in any form or by any means, electronic or mechanical, including photocopying, microfilm and recording, or by any information storage and retrieval system, without permission in writing from the publisher. Printed in the United States of America.

The development, preparation, and publication of this work has been undertaken with great care. However, the publisher, employees, editors, and agents of The Haworth Press and all imprints of The Haworth Press, Inc., including The Haworth Medical Press® and Pharmaceutical Products Press®, are not responsible for any errors contained herein or for consequences that may ensue from use of materials or information contained in this work. Opinions expressed by the author(s) are not necessarily those of The Haworth Press, Inc. With regard to case studies, identities and circumstances of individuals discussed herein have been changed to protect confidentiality. Any resemblance to actual persons, living or dead, is entirely coincidental.

Cover design by Marylouise E. Doyle

Library of Congress Cataloging-in-Publication Data

Handbook for pharmacy educators : getting adjusted as a new pharmacy faculty member / Shane P. Desselle, Dana P. Hammer, editors.
    p. ; cm.
  "Co-published simultaneously as Journal of pharmacy teaching, volume 9, number 1, 2002."
  Includes bibliographical references and index.
  ISBN 0-7890-1986-8 (hard : alk. paper)–ISBN 0-7890-1987-6 (pbk. : alk. paper)
  1. Pharmacy–Study and teaching–Handbooks, manuals, etc.
[DNLM: 1. Education, Pharmacy–methods. QV 18 H2355 2002] I. Desselle, Shane P. II. Hammer, Dana P. III. Journal of pharmacy teaching.
RS101.H355 2002
615'.1'0711–dc21
                                                     2002005461

Indexing, Abstracting & Website/Internet Coverage

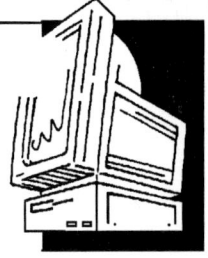

This section provides you with a list of major indexing & abstracting services. That is to say, each service began covering this periodical during the year noted in the right column. Most Websites which are listed below have indicated that they will either post, disseminate, compile, archive, cite or alert their own Website users with research-based content from this work. (This list is as current as the copyright date of this publication.)

Abstracting, Website/Indexing Coverage......... Year When Coverage Began

- *CNPIEC Reference Guide: Chinese National Directory of Foreign Periodicals* 1995

- *Educational Research Abstracts (ERA) (online database) <www.tandf.co.uk>*....................................... 2002

- *FINDEX <www.publist.com>*............................. 1999

- *International Pharmaceutical Abstracts*..................... 1989

- *Pharmacy Business* 1993

- *Referativnyi Zhurnal (Abstracts Journal of the All-Russian Institute of Scientific and Technical Information-in Russian)* . 1990

- *SwetsNet <www.swetsnet.com>*............................ 2002

- *Technical Education & Training Abstracts* 1993

Special Bibliographic Notes related to special journal issues (separates) and indexing/abstracting:

- indexing/abstracting services in this list will also cover material in any "separate" that is co-published simultaneously with Haworth's special thematic journal issue or DocuSerial. Indexing/abstracting usually covers material at the article/chapter level.
- monographic co-editions are intended for either non-subscribers or libraries which intend to purchase a second copy for their circulating collections.
- monographic co-editions are reported to all jobbers/wholesalers/approval plans. The source journal is listed as the "series" to assist the prevention of duplicate purchasing in the same manner utilized for books-in-series.
- to facilitate user/access services all indexing/abstracting services are encouraged to utilize the co-indexing entry note indicated at the bottom of the first page of each article/chapter/contribution.
- this is intended to assist a library user of any reference tool (whether print, electronic, online, or CD-ROM) to locate the monographic version if the library has purchased this version but not a subscription to the source journal.
- individual articles/chapters in any Haworth publication are also available through the Haworth Document Delivery Service (HDDS).

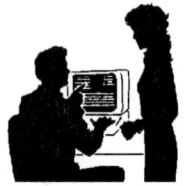

Handbook for Pharmacy Educators: Getting Adjusted As a New Pharmacy Faculty Member

CONTENTS

Introduction   1
   Shane P. Desselle
   Dana P. Hammer

Establishing Equilibrium in the Pretenure Years:
   A Chemist's Perspective in a School of Pharmacy   9
   John M. Rimoldi

Persistence and Patience–Necessities for New Faculty
   Members: Experiences of a First-Year Pharmacy Practice
   Faculty Member at a Public University   19
   Nanette Bultemeier

New Challenges, New Opportunities: Perspective
   of a New Faculty Member   35
   Scott K. Stolte

And You Think Your Job Stinks? Think Again:
   Every Cloud Does Have a Silver Lining   47
   Gireesh V. Gupchup

Life and Times of a New Social and Administrative
   Sciences Faculty Member   61
   Ana C. Quiñones

Succeeding in Academe–Self-Management and Passion   73
   Lon N. Larson

Index   85

∞ ALL PHARMACEUTICAL PRODUCTS PRESS BOOKS AND JOURNALS ARE PRINTED ON CERTIFIED ACID-FREE PAPER

ABOUT THE EDITORS

Shane P. Desselle, Ph.D., is Assistant Director of Pharmacy Administration and Director of Assessment and Educational Strategies at Duquesne University. He hails from a small town in Louisiana and received his B.S. in Pharmacy and Ph.D. in Pharmacy Administration from Northeast Louisiana University. He has practice experience in both community and hospital pharmacy. Dr. Desselle is involved in the use of psychometric techniques for applied research purposes, including the development of a scale to access consumer satisfaction with their prescription drug coverage and the construction of a template by which to conduct performance appraisals of community pharmacy technicians. He is also engaged in research aimed at measuring the use of persuasion in direct-to-consumer prescription drug advertising and assessing the "scientific progress" of the social and administrative pharmaceutical sciences. Dr. Desselle serves on the editorial advisory boards of the *Journal of the American Pharmaceutical Association* and the *Journal of Managed Care Pharmacy*. He has published over 20 papers in the past five years. He teaches classes at Duquesne on American health care systems, health care economics, social and behavioral issues in pharmacy practice, and research methods in pharmacy administration.

Dana P. Hammer, Ph.D., is Director of the Bracken Pharmaceutical Care Learning Center and the UW Community Pharmacy Residency Program for the University of Washington School of Pharmacy. Dr. Hammer received her B.S. in Pharmacy from Oregon State University, worked two years in hospital and community independent pharmacies, then returned to school to earn her master's degree and Ph.D. from Purdue University School of Pharmacy. In her graduate coursework, Dr. Hammer focused on education, sociology and psychology as they relate to pharmacy and other health professions' education. Her research involves assessment of students' educational outcomes and professional development and she has published numerous articles on these topics. She has served as a faculty member for two AACP Institutes and has presented faculty development workshops on student assessment, professionalism and active learning techniques to faculty at several pharmacy schools and national conferences. She also serves on the editorial board of the *Journal of Pharmacy Teaching*. Dr. Hammer has won several awards for teaching, innovations in teaching and education, educational research and service to the pharmacy profession.

Introduction

Shane P. Desselle
Dana P. Hammer

A recent Ph.D. graduate was ready to begin his first day as a new faculty member. It was a bitterly cold morning in New York City as he awaited the "F" train at the Forest Hills, Queens station in hope that it would expeditiously transport him to the Arnold & Marie Schwartz College of Pharmacy and Health Sciences of Long Island University in downtown Brooklyn. One and one-half hours later, he arrived at the foot of the gated campus and was greeted by a security guard who looked at him in astonishment. "Hi, I'm Shane Desselle," he sheepishly spoke, "a new member of the faculty in the School of Pharmacy. Can you let me in? I don't have an ID or a key to my office, yet." He responded, "The university is closed today. Didn't you know–with yesterday's blizzard and all?" So this eager new faculty member turned right back around with briefcase in hand, and journeyed back to Forest Hills. This time, however, the trip back was only 1 hour and 15 minutes.

This new faculty member's second attempt to get started at his new job was much more fruitful. He got inside the gate and even into his office this time. Waiting for him were the desk, filing cabinet, and lavish

---

Shane P. Desselle, Ph.D., is Assistant Professor of Pharmacy Administration and Director of Assessment and Educational Strategies at the Mylan School of Pharmacy, Duquesne University, Pittsburgh, PA 15282 (E-mail: desselle@duq.edu). Dana P. Hammer, Ph.D., is Director, Bracken Pharmaceutical Care Learning Center and UW Community Pharmacy Residency Program, University of Washington School of Pharmacy, Box 357630, Seattle, WA 98195-7630 (E-mail: dphammer@u.washington.edu).

[Haworth co-indexing entry note]: "Introduction." Desselle, Shane P., and Dana P. Hammer. Co-published simultaneously in *Journal of Pharmacy Teaching* (Pharmaceutical Products Press, an imprint of The Haworth Press, Inc.) Vol. 9, No. 1, 2002, pp. 1-7; and: *Handbook for Pharmacy Educators: Getting Adjusted As a New Pharmacy Faculty Member* (ed: Shane P. Desselle and Dana P. Hammer) Pharmaceutical Products Press, an imprint of The Haworth Press, Inc., 2002, pp. 1-7. Single or multiple copies of this article are available for a fee from The Haworth Document Delivery Service [1-800-HAWORTH, 9:00 a.m. - 5:00 p.m. (EST). E-mail address: getinfo@haworthpressinc.com].

© 2002 by The Haworth Press, Inc. All rights reserved.   *1 executive chair he had ordered. Not waiting for him, though, were a computer, paper, pens, or any faint idea of how to get started. Then it dawned on this new academic, how autonomous a faculty member's job is. This eager Ph.D. literally sat in his chair, staring at the walls, out the window, and at the department secretary for nearly an hour. "Well, what do I do, now?" he thought. "There are no instructions here." He then figured that whatever he was supposed to do, however he was supposed to do it, he had better get started because in just two more weeks he was going to be coursemaster and sole instructor for three different courses–none of which he had ever taught, two of which were new in the curriculum, and one of which had no existing syllabus or notes for him to use. He then proceeded to purchase a notebook from the bookstore and began developing syllabi and writing lectures.*

How humbling this and other experiences throughout a new faculty member's first year or two in academe can be, especially when compared to how a new graduate feels just a few short weeks prior to beginning a job. Taking the stage, being hooded, and being welcomed into the ranks of the "truly educated" is an uplifting experience. Families and friends travel hours to bask in the pride at the attainment of the highest degree that universities have to offer. But the pride and the celebrations, while remembered forever, may not adequately squelch the stress associated with beginning a new academic position.

No matter how well your major advisor conditions you and whether or not you engaged in some teaching while a doctoral student, resident, or fellow, you are certainly not fully prepared to assume the roles and responsibilities of a faculty position immediately upon completing your postgraduate education. Suddenly, after years of sitting in desks taking in vast amounts of information, the shoe is on the other foot. In just a few short years between our undergraduate education and that first day on the new academic job, we seem to forget how students, especially entry-level degree students, think and learn. Having completed graduate study and obtained such a wealth of knowledge in a very specific and concentrated area, we come to think of what we know as "old hat." We underestimate the knowledge we have obtained in this specific area yet overestimate our general knowledge. This is why many new faculty members struggle–we assume students are well versed in our knowledge, and even worse, we assume that they are as interested as we are in the subject matter that we teach. The medicinal chemist assumes that students share the same enthusiasm he or she does about structure-activity relationships, and the social and administrative scientist assumes that if he or she casually mentions the Health Belief Model to students that students already know what he or she is talking about. Conversely, we may enter the academic institution and relationships with administrators and fellow colleagues thinking that we know far more than we actually do.

This is one of the reasons we embarked on compiling these manuscripts. We hope that from this issue stakeholders–new faculty members, more experienced faculty members, division chairs, deans, and administrators–can glean some ideas that will assist junior faculty members in launching productive and successful careers. Junior faculty members, after all, are the educators, researchers, and academic administrators of the future. Their role in shaping universities with their new ideas, their fresh approach, and their scholarly endeavors is paramount. Every new faculty member is going to stumble, and nothing in this issue or any other source is going to change that; however, if the creative energies of the new faculty member are overly obstructed, then not only does that individual suffer, but the school of pharmacy and the institution do as well.

There is little doubt that the expectations for faculty in the U.S. have been rising. Faculty in traditionally research-oriented institutions are expected to teach more and teach well, while those employed in teaching, tuition-driven institutions are expected to generate more scholarship and secure at least some external funding. Many new pharmacy faculty are strapped with expectations that they receive very good to excellent teaching evaluations from students in addition to National Institutes of Health (NIH) funding in order for them to be tenured and promoted to the associate professor level. The difficulties can be even greater for females, who have demonstrated a greater propensity to leave their institutions prior to a tenure decision and are more likely to be denied tenure (1-3). Nonwhite newer faculty also encounter the additional obstacles of marginalization and insensitivity (4-6). Indeed, it has been demonstrated that stress is an increasingly significant problem for these and many new faculty members (7).

Some of the specific stressful factors for new faculty have been studied and include "not enough time," inadequate feedback and recognition, unrealistic expectations, lack of collegiality, and difficulty in balancing work and life outside of work (8). For pharmacy faculty (not necessarily new), the 5 most stressful situations from a list of 31 were securing financial support for research, having sufficient time to keep abreast of current developments in individuals' research fields, feeling that their workload is so heavy that all tasks cannot possibly be completed during the normal work day, imposing excessively high self-expectations, and attending meetings that take up too much time (9). A more recent study of junior faculty in schools of pharmacy reported that:

- Respondents were ambivalent with regard to their satisfaction of the teaching, research, and service roles.
- Respondents were most satisfied with their teaching roles and least satisfied with their research roles.
- Females were significantly less satisfied with their roles than their male counterparts.
- Those employed in private schools were significantly less satisfied than those employed by public universities.
- Those working in schools six years or less in existence were significantly less satisfied than those working in schools in existence more than six years (10).

Other studies have been conducted on some of the individual aforementioned factors. When examining the balance between work and personal life, one study reported that half of the respondents surveyed reported a positive "spillover" effect between their professional and personal lives, while half also reported stress in trying to balance time and commitment to family with career aspirations. A higher degree of this spillover is more likely to be experienced by academicians than the general population (11). A study of the effects of work, nonwork, and role conflict on the overall life satisfaction of pharmacy faculty found that respondents were only moderately satisfied with their lives and identified being married, receiving social support from spouses or mates, and socializing with friends as nonwork influences that were related to life satisfaction. Many of these same influences were related to role conflict (12).

Differences in job satisfaction between first-year faculty and more senior faculty also have been studied. Findings showed that more senior faculty reported optimistic and enthusiastic beginnings, but, over time, work stress increased and job satisfaction deteriorated. Budget restrictions and less resource availability were seen as being detrimental to career development. First-year faculty desired more assistance than they received in adjusting to their new setting and in establishing themselves as researchers and teachers, a condition particularly strong in female faculty. Eighty-two percent of faculty, after their first year, indicated a likelihood of seeking jobs with other universities within the next year

(13). With regard to teaching, one study suggested that new faculty teach "defensively": they emphasize content over student involvement, rarely seek or receive collegial help, and resent teaching as an activity that undermines scholarship (14). However, another study showed that as new faculty matured into their careers they spent less time on teaching preparation, teaching was increasingly perceived as more satisfying and less stressful than research, an increased amount of time was spent on research, and there was increased stress about research productivity and increased perception of work stress (15).

An additional challenge facing new pharmacy faculty is the understanding they must gain of pharmacy's other disciplines, which are also involved in educating the entry-level student. Some pharmacy faculty did not receive their undergraduate education in pharmacy. Moreover, the disciplines in pharmacy are unique, and the experiences shared by new faculty in each of these areas, while having some commonality, can be quite disparate. In addition to the obvious differences in the types of courses that are taught and research endeavors that are initiated, the disciplines in pharmacy are different by their being newer versus older, pure versus applied, biological versus nonbiological. The disciplines vary, then, in the degree to which they have achieved consensus on issues to research, appropriate research methodologies, and strategies used in teaching (16). This variation of having achieved consensus or "scientific progress" has implications in how these faculty members view teaching and research and ultimately how they handle stress and adjust to their roles (17).

Differences among disciplines is one of the primary reasons this compilation is structured the way that it is. It features five junior faculty authors, two each from the clinical and social and administrative sciences and one from the basic sciences, representing diversity in ethnicity, gender, and type of institution where employed, sharing their experiences from their first few years in academe. They provide their insight on what worked and did not work for them as they launched their academic careers. This is followed by commentary and observations from a highly accomplished senior faculty member.

A growing body of literature has been devoted to recommendations for faculty development programs and the success and retention of new faculty members (3, 18-21). This compilation is meant to add to this body of work and to share the specific experiences of six pharmacy faculty members. It is hoped that the insights gained from these papers will prove useful to junior and senior pharmacy faculty members alike.

REFERENCES

1. Tack MW, Patitu CL. Faculty job satisfaction: Women and minorities in peril. ASHE-ERIC Higher Education Report No. 4. Washington, DC: George Washington University; 1992.
2. Dwyer MM, Flynn AA, Inmann PS. Differential progress of women faculty: Status 1980-1990. In: Higher education: Handbook of theory and research. Vol. 7. Smart JC, ed. New York: Agathon; 1991:173-222.
3. Sandler BR. Success and survival strategies for women faculty members. Am J Pharm Educ. 1993; 57:58-67.
4. Johnsrud LK. Women and minority faculty experiences: Defining and responding to diverse realities. In: Building a diverse faculty. New directions for teaching and learning. No. 53. Gainen J, Boice R, eds. San Francisco: Jossey-Bass; 1993.
5. Boice R. Early turning points in professorial careers of women and minorities. In: Building a diverse faculty. New directions for teaching and learning. No. 53. Gainen J, Boice R, eds. San Francisco: Jossey-Bass; 1993.
6. Garza H. Second-class academics: Chicano/Latino faculty in U.S. universities. In: Building a diverse faculty. New directions for teaching and learning. No. 53. Gainen J, Boice R, eds. San Francisco: Jossey-Bass; 1993.
7. Menges RJ. Dilemmas of newly hired faculty. In: Faculty in new jobs: A guide to settling in, becoming established, and building institutional support. Menges RJ, ed. San Francisco: Jossey-Bass; 1999:19-38.
8. Sorcinelli MD. New and junior faculty stress: Research and responses. New directions for teaching and learning. No. 50. San Francisco: Jossey-Bass; 1992: 27-37.
9. Wolfgang AP. Job stress and dissatisfaction among school of pharmacy faculty members. Am J Pharm Educ. 1993; 57:215-21.
10. Latif DA, Grillo JA. Satisfaction of junior faculty with academic role functions. Am J Pharm Educ. 2001; 65:137-43.
11. Near JP, Sorcinelli MD. Work and life away from work: Predictors of faculty satisfaction. Res Higher Educ. 1986; 25:77-94.
12. Nair KV, Gaither CA. Effects of work, nonwork, and role conflict on the overall life satisfaction of pharmacy faculty. Am J Pharm Educ. 1999; 63:1-11.
13. Sorcinelli MD, Billings DA. The career development of pretenure faculty: An institutional study. Paper presented at the Annual Meeting of the American Educational Research Association, Atlanta, GA, 1992.
14. Boice R. New faculty as teachers. J Higher Educ. 1991; 62(2):150-73.
15. Olsen D, Sorcinelli MD. The pretenure years: A longitudinal perspective. New directions for teaching and learning. No. 50. San Francisco: Jossey-Bass; 1992: 15-25.
16. Biglan A. The characteristics of subject matter in different academic areas. J Appl Psychol. 1973; 57:195-203.
17. Braxton JM, Hargens LL. Variation among academic disciplines: Analytical frameworks and research. In: Higher education: Handbook of theory and research. Vol. 11. Smart JC, ed. New York: Agathon; 1996:1-46.
18. Boice R. Quick starters: New faculty who succeed. Effective practices for improving teaching. New directions for teaching and learning. Vol. 48. San Francisco: Jossey-Bass; 1991:111-21.

19. Boice R. The new faculty member: Supporting and fostering professional development. San Francisco: Jossey-Bass; 1992.
20. Boice R. New faculty involvement for women and minorities. Res Higher Educ. 1993; 34:291-341.
21. Sorcinelli MD. Effective approaches to new faculty development. J Counsel Develop. 1994; 72(5):74-9.

Establishing Equilibrium in the Pretenure Years: A Chemist's Perspective in a School of Pharmacy

John M. Rimoldi

The invitation to participate in this special issue regarding new faculty in pharmacy couldn't have come at a more auspicious time, since I recently concentrated the initial five years of my academic career (all the essence and substance fitting in a three-ring binder) in the submission of my tenure and promotion dossier. My intentions in writing this manuscript are not rooted in pontificating about the tenure process, but as I begin to consider its impact and effects on my academic freedom, expectations, and attitudes in these tenure-track years, I have come to the realization that *it is this single process that disenchants the majority of new faculty.* My opinion is shared by a commentary concerning a recent survey of faculty opinion, conducted in the fall of 1996, that revealed a striking 38% of respondents were disappointed with the current tenure system–that figure approaching 43% among female faculty (1). It has been stated that "gaining tenure–or the fear of not gaining it–is a significant intrinsic motivator for faculty" (2). Since tenure lies at the

---

John M. Rimoldi, Ph.D., is Assistant Professor of Medicinal Chemistry and Research Associate Professor in the Research Institute of Pharmaceutical Sciences, School of Pharmacy, University of Mississippi, University, MS 38677 (E-mail: jrimoldi@olemiss.edu).

[Haworth co-indexing entry note]: "Establishing Equilibrium in the Pretenure Years: A Chemist's Perspective in a School of Pharmacy." Rimoldi, John M. Co-published simultaneously in *Journal of Pharmacy Teaching* (Pharmaceutical Products Press, an imprint of The Haworth Press, Inc.) Vol. 9, No. 1, 2002, pp. 9-17; and: *Handbook for Pharmacy Educators: Getting Adjusted As a New Pharmacy Faculty Member* (ed: Shane P. Desselle and Dana P. Hammer) Pharmaceutical Products Press, an imprint of The Haworth Press, Inc., 2002, pp. 9-17. Single or multiple copies of this article are available for a fee from The Haworth Document Delivery Service [1-800-HAWORTH, 9:00 a.m. - 5:00 p.m. (EST). E-mail address: getinfo@haworthpressinc.com].

© 2002 by The Haworth Press, Inc. All rights reserved.

crux of differentiating most junior faculty from the rest of the academy, I am of the opinion that the pretenure process shapes our decision-making processes as we strive to establish tripartite excellence as academicians and will eventually affect the way we "do business" in the inaugural years. In this tone, I will attempt to share some lessons learned from the perspective of one who entered the pharmacy academic community devoid of any formal pharmacy training or expertise.

The University of Mississippi is a public institution with campuses in Oxford (main), Jackson, Tupelo, and Southaven, Mississippi. It houses the state's only pharmacy school and medical school, and has a total student enrollment of 12,500. The School of Pharmacy's administrative structure is rather complex, with six academic departments (Pharmacy Practice, Medicinal Chemistry, Pharmaceutics, Pharmacology, Pharmacognosy, Pharmacy Administration), the Research Institute of Pharmaceutical Sciences (research activities conducted through the National Center for Natural Products Research and Environmental and Community Health Research), and a Center for Pharmaceutical Marketing and Management, all under the school's administrative umbrella. Most academic full-time faculty members are granted joint appointments in the Research Institute. The School of Pharmacy is located on the Oxford campus with the exception of the Department of Pharmacy Practice, which is mainly located on the Jackson Campus (two hours south of Oxford). Communication between the two campuses has improved over the last few years due to enhancement of technology but remains less than desirable due to distance factors.

One of the strengths of the School of Pharmacy is the academic departmental structure, which allows for new faculty and graduate students to maintain an "identity" within their discipline. This is in direct contrast to institutions that have consolidated diverse departments into a single pharmaceutical sciences division. I represent 1 of 6 faculty in the Department of Medicinal Chemistry, with a graduate student enrollment of approximately 15-20 students, similar in size to the other 4 basic science departments in the school. Undergraduate students are admitted formally into the School of Pharmacy under the B.S. in Pharmaceutical Sciences degree program. Students in this program may choose one of six tracks to follow, each preparatory for a different career path. For example, undergraduate students in their P3 year may elect to continue in the Medicinal Chemistry Track in the P4 year, which would comprise courses in advanced medicinal chemistry and associated laboratory experience. Students completing the track in medicinal chemistry have opportunities to seek employment in the pharmaceutical industry as B.S. degree scientists or to seek an advanced degree in a graduate program. The majority of students elect to continue in the general pharmacy track en route to the professional Pharm.D. degree. The School of Pharmacy has recently (1996) instituted the Pharm.D. degree as the sole practice degree and also offers a postbaccalaureate Doctor of Pharmacy for practicing pharmacists who wish to supplement their professional education and further develop their clinical skills. Advanced degrees (M.S., Ph.D.) are offered in each of the basic science departments; graduates of the Department of Medicinal Chemistry traditionally seek employment in the pharmaceutical industry, academic or industrial postdoctoral appointments, or academic appointments.

Having a background in the chemical sciences with a Ph.D. degree in organic chemistry and related postdoctoral experience in bioorganic chemistry, my expectations formed through these training experiences were first reckoned in light of the realities of the academic role and workload. Most new faculty members leave graduate school or a postdoctoral appointment ill-prepared to assume new and immediate responsibilities of teaching, research, and service. After arriving on campus, one must adjust to an academic climate with different cultures, missions, and expectations from the one left behind. This period of readjustment has been commonly referred to as the encounter phase and may last up to three years (3). A key task at this phase is role definition, which involves clarifying responsibilities, establishing priorities, and allocating time productively (4). Diminishing the time spent in the encounter phase is fundamental to increasing scholarly productivity in the pretenure period. This may be accomplished largely with a formal faculty mentoring program. Although I was informally mentored into academics by my postdoctoral advisor, I was first introduced to the concept of faculty mentoring through the American Association of Colleges of Pharmacy (AACP)-driven Mentoring Program, launched by the Section of Teachers of Medicinal Chemistry in 1996. This inaugural initiative matched senior faculty (one external mentor, one internal mentor) with nontenured faculty (protégé) to facilitate the protégé's success in teaching and research responsibilities. Although the dynamics of faculty mentoring have long been considered a "natural" phenomenon that occurs without a procedural requisite, having a structured program is fundamental for a variety of reasons. New faculty members are particularly susceptible to the negative pressures of new academic assignments, lack of social support networks, and exposure to department/school/university discord and weaknesses not immediately apparent during the interview. Active mentorship is especially important in these circumstances because, traditionally, new faculty members are passive in seeking help that may be misinterpreted as a sign of weakness. I profit from having mentors with excellent listening skills, positive collegial attitudes, and a firm commitment to my professional development. A formal mentoring program also increases protégé accountability to the mentor and, ultimately, to the university. Long-term career planning is facilitated, stress levels are reduced, and collegiality between senior and junior faculty is enhanced. This process should mirror the mentoring process that occurs habitually between a graduate student and a faculty advisor. I will comment on several tangible benefits reaped from this mentoring process in later sections.

For the mentoring process to operate efficiently, collegiality among faculty members at all levels must be fostered. The collegial atmosphere intra- and interdepartmentally at the university has been outstanding; this climate was prominent during the interview process and has not changed substantially over the last five years. Collegiality cannot be taken lightly and must be continually cultivated in a profession that is inherently multifaceted and highly autonomous. The "met expectations" hypothesis predicts "that when an individual's [job] expectations–whatever they are–are not substantially met, his propensity to withdrawal should increase" (5). Most of my research and teaching collaborations have occurred by virtue of the collegial environment in the school and, ultimately, have lead to greater job satisfaction and increased productivity. A collegial climate is also fundamental to provide students (graduate and undergraduate) with examples of solid professional relationships and attitudes at the professorial level.

It is difficult, but not impossible, to strike a proper balance between the demands of maintaining a rigorous research agenda and the recent calls for a renewed dedication to teaching (6). A common grievance for most new faculty is that there is only a limited amount of time that one can devote to research activities given other faculty time allocations, particularly in a public research-oriented institution. Faculty time expenditures have great influence on faculty research output, which affects retention, promotion, compensation, and peer recognition, especially considering the current reward structure, in which "published research is the common currency of academic achievement" (7, 8). However, increased time allocation to research activities is not necessarily correlated with increased research productivity. For example, my first semester in academe was dedicated principally to writing grant applications, setting up my laboratory, and becoming accustomed to the new university structure. I fervently scrambled the first year, targeting extramural agencies with funding interests similar to my research interests, even if the similarities were scant at best. I spent more time trying to secure funding than maturing my research projects and interests. After having some immediate success at securing external funding within the first year, I was faced with the responsibility of managing those grants and fulfilling the specific aims outlined in the projects. I then had grant dollars secured to purchase commodities and equipment and to support a graduate student, but I did not have any full-time graduate students under my direct supervision until year three of my academic appointment. Coupled with a start-up package that was not sufficient to hire a postdoctoral research associate or technician, these initial grants did not produce the outcomes I had envisioned. Research *timing* was more critical than the *time* available in this instance. Although I consider these events part of the professional development experience, they can be injurious during the pretenure years. Rebounding from such experiences is difficult but was enabled by continual mentoring and advice by seasoned faculty. The same timing issues will undoubtedly surface in the domain of teaching.

I was initially introduced to the departmental teaching activities at a gradual, but deliberate, pace over the last five years. This is an exemplary method of faculty professional development for new assistant professors, insofar as it enabled me to devote dedicated time to research activities at the onset, and it progressively introduced me to the methods of instruction in a school of pharmacy. Gradual increases in teaching responsibilities allowed me to spend time observing my colleagues in the classroom and provided me with opportunities to develop my own course material. Having a background in organic chemistry, it was not an easy task to enter a professional curriculum and be responsible for teaching and training future pharmacists. I expended a great deal of time learning the "language" of a pharmacist and learning how to teach this new language. I also had to divorce myself from trying to force-feed organic chemistry at the undergraduate level (known to produce "chemophobia") and to focus on teaching pharmacists the influence that medicinal chemistry has on pharmacy (9). I also reserved time for developing new graduate-level courses in our curriculum.

Instruction at the graduate level in medicinal chemistry has been extremely enjoyable, particularly since it has kept me current with advances in the field and allowed for the refinement of my teaching methods at a more advanced level. Moreover, our department operates on the tenet that each faculty member is given an opportunity to select courses to instruct based on subdiscipline expertise and semester load. Teaching loads and obligations in a school of pharmacy are minimal in comparison to most nonprofessional degree programs like chemistry. The university has created an extensive support environment for teaching by providing faculty with state-of-the-art instructional technologies, teaching workshops, and faculty-to-faculty forums on pedagogical issues. The School of Pharmacy also has been instrumental in providing new faculty with resources and funds to enhance instructional frameworks in each academic department. For example, the School of Pharmacy has provided travel funds for faculty to attend AACP meetings, equipped classrooms with state-of-the-art technology, and instituted a School of Pharmacy Faculty Instructional Innovations Award.

Although the academic support structure is in place, it is not clear if the university's administration weighs excellence in teaching as heavily as excellence in research in the tenure and promotion process. Wolverton argues, "Rewards for research and publications, and punishments for failure to accomplish these, are well defined and substantial; but rewards (the granting of tenure or promotion, for example) for good teaching remain limited" (2). Intrinsic rewards abound (teaching satisfaction, positive student/peer feedback, self-evaluation and assessments), but external rewards are few. Although philosophies such as these may sound the gloom and doom alarm, there are methods one can employ to try to establish equity between teaching and research during the tenure and promotion process. One path I chose to take involved the creation of a teaching portfolio, which established an opportunity for my colleagues and the administration to review my teaching in a more objective and substantial manner.

My external mentor was the first to suggest that I consider creating a teaching portfolio; he provided me with a portfolio template in addition to advice concerning its content. Although discussions concerning the importance of creating teaching portfolios have occurred at both the school and university level at the University of Mississippi, efforts to adopt this practice globally have not been pursued aggressively. Nonetheless, I constructed my teaching portfolio using a combination of two templates (10, 11). My portfolio included evidence of teaching excellence, containing particulars such as new course development, course revisions, innovative methods of instruction, semester course loads and size, graduate and undergraduate advising (in the form of research or academic advising), graduate student theses/dissertation committee service, and other factors that contribute overall to professional development. Another component included assessment and evaluation (students, peer, and self), which is critical and takes time to construct. Included in the portfolio was supplemental documentation (syllabi, student evaluations, peer evaluations, and published and communicated contributions to teaching) in the form of an appendix.

I also had an opportunity to restructure my teaching philosophy to accommodate the changes I made to my methods and styles of instruction. Before entering academe, my teaching philosophy was shaped by what I had observed in the classroom (i.e., based on my observations of effective teachers from a student perspective). However, after several years of teaching, my perspective reflected my own experiences, from which I created four fundamental principles (PROF: Passion, Rapport, Organization, Fairness) based on the tenet "by example"; these principles serve as the foundation of my teaching philosophy. I discovered that I design instruction so that the students actively use specific intellectual skills to analyze various dimensions of course content. This is particularly important in a basic science course like medicinal chemistry. Students stand to learn more as a result of developing their intellectual skills, abilities, standards, and disciplines. They have the opportunity to assess their own work and learn how to assess the work of others. The overall process of portfolio development was extremely rewarding. I would encourage all new faculty to begin to assemble a teaching portfolio early in the academic pretenure process. It cannot be constructed in one sitting, but must evolve with time and be continually remodeled and shaped to be effective.

Service adopts different forms at all levels of academe. The current academic reward structure must be broadened to include measures and outcomes of service productivity, although this is unlikely to occur anytime soon. The question has been posed, "Is it advisable to decline requests for service, or will this be viewed negatively?" (7). This conflict abounds in the initial years, where the "just say no" policy for service may have immediate individual benefits in terms of time allocation but be detrimental in the long term if one is labeled as noncollegial or a nonplayer. The discord places new faculty in an ethical bind and limits faculty decision making to "whatever is best for tenure." Although new faculty members are likely to enhance and broaden the scope of the missions of the department, school, university, profession, and community through the service component, the current reward structure argues against time allocations for service activities. Equity in service has been steady within our department during my initial years but has shifted with the recent departure of one faculty member and the movement of three faculty members to interim administrative positions. Does a faculty member "just say no" to service functions in light of these particular circumstances? Creamer states, "The profile of faculty across this country has remained so stubbornly homogenous because of the reluctance to relinquish traditional measures of faculty productivity. A narrow definition of what constitutes a contribution to knowledge represents only a fragment of academic discourse, and it awards the privilege of an authoritative voice to only a few scholars" (12).

After an evaluation of my initial five years, it became obvious that I had overcommitted to service activities during the pretenure period, perhaps to my disadvantage. In retrospect, I would argue against committing to an inordinate number of service activities, but there are several that I thoroughly enjoy and have found to overlap well with other scholarly activities. Serving as a manuscript reviewer, a member on a grant application review panel (study section), and providing professional society leadership have allowed me to give back to my profession, promote the visibility of our department, keep current with new advances in the field, and establish new professional relationships.

In light of the tripartite academic responsibilities, how does a new faculty member know he/she is on track? Our university adopted, many years ago, a yearly review in the form of an activity report for all faculty members (including tenured faculty); it is especially valuable during the pretenure years. These activity reports contain evidence of productivity in all arenas for each year of appointment. The tenured faculty members in each representative department review the new faculty members, and a comprehensive written evaluation is provided each year. My department chairman extends this practice by having a one-on-one meeting with me following the departmental review to discuss the review in terms of progression. In this capacity, I am made fully aware of my standing each year during the pretenure phase and can implement changes that are necessary to improve my progress.

So how does one establish equilibrium in the pretenure years? I think the answer to this question varies markedly with the type of faculty appointment (clinical, research, teaching). However, it can be established with a department, school, and university dedicated to a mission centered on the professional development of new faculty members, rewarding them for all areas of achievement (teaching, research, and service) when warranted. Tenure and promotion are indeed part of the reward system and should reflect the tripartite role charged to each of us in the academy.

REFERENCES

1. O'Neil RM. Academic freedom: Revolutionary change or business as usual? Rev Higher Educ. 1998; 21:257-65.
2. Wolverton M. Treading the tenure-track tightrope: Finding balance between research excellence and quality teaching. Innovative Higher Educ. 1998; 23:61-79.
3. Feldman DC. The multiple socialization of organization members. Acad Manage Rev. 1981; 6:308-18.
4. Olsen D, Crawford LA. A five-year study of junior faculty expectations about their work. Rev Higher Educ. 1998; 22:39-54.
5. Porter LW, Steers RM. Organizational, work, and personal factors in employee turnover and absenteeism. Psychol Bull. 1993; 80:151-76.
6. Cole J. Balancing acts: Dilemmas of choice facing research universities. In: The research university in a time of discontent. Cole J, Barber E, Graubard S, eds. Baltimore: Johns Hopkins University Press; 1994:1-36.
7. Bellas ML, Toutkoushian RK. Faculty time allocations and research productivity: Gender, race and family effects. Rev Higher Educ. 1999; 22:367-90.
8. Rau W, Baker P. The organized contradictions of academe: Barriers facing the next academic revolution. Teach Sociol. 1989; 17:165-75.
9. Eddy RM. Chemophobia in the college classroom: Extent, sources, and student characteristics. J Chem Educ. 2000; 77:514-7.
10. Lemke T. Personal communication. University of Houston School of Pharmacy.
11. Barry K. Guidelines for writing a teaching portfolio. Professional Development Centre, Edith Cowan University, 1997 [resource on World Wide Web]. URL: http://www.ecu.edu.au/eddev/tchport/tchcont.htm. Available from Internet.
12. Creamer L. Assessing faculty publication productivity: Issues of equity. ASHE-ERIC Higher Education Report Number 26. Washington, DC: ASHE-ERIC/George Washington University Graduate School of Education and Human Development, 1998.

Persistence and Patience– Necessities for New Faculty Members: Experiences of a First-Year Pharmacy Practice Faculty Member at a Public University

Nanette Bultemeier

INTRODUCTION

In my desk drawer at the office I keep a small piece of paper from a personal journal that I had used to jot my thoughts as I was completing my application to pharmacy school. "Ten-year goal–once I am established, I'd like to further my education in such a way that I will be able to integrate my knowledge as a pharmacist with my skills outside of pharmacy and apply them to a related field such as education. . . ."

After graduating with my Pharm.D., I continued my education by completing a pharmacy practice residency and a primary care residency. I was hired as an Assistant Professor of Pharmacy Practice at Oregon State University about 2 years ago, in August 1999. It has been ten years since I wrote my ten-year goal as a first-year college student.

I have been asked to share my experiences as a new faculty member

---

Nanette Bultemeier, Pharm.D., is Assistant Professor of Pharmacy Practice at Oregon State University College of Pharmacy, 840 SW Gaines Street, GH 212, Portland, OR 97201 (E-mail: bultemei@ohsu.edu).

[Haworth co-indexing entry note]: "Persistence and Patience–Necessities for New Faculty Members: Experiences of a First-Year Pharmacy Practice Faculty Member at a Public University." Bultemeier, Nanette. Co-published simultaneously in *Journal of Pharmacy Teaching* (Pharmaceutical Products Press, an imprint of The Haworth Press, Inc.) Vol. 9, No. 1, 2002, pp. 19-33; and: *Handbook for Pharmacy Educators: Getting Adjusted As a New Pharmacy Faculty Member* (ed: Shane P. Desselle and Dana P. Hammer) Pharmaceutical Products Press, an imprint of The Haworth Press, Inc., 2002, pp. 19-33. Single or multiple copies of this article are available for a fee from The Haworth Document Delivery Service [1-800-HAWORTH, 9:00 a.m. - 5:00 p.m. (EST). E-mail address: getinfo@haworthpressinc.com].

© 2002 by The Haworth Press, Inc. All rights reserved.

so that current and future new faculty members, senior colleagues, and pharmacy school administrators can gain insight into this important transition. A brief description of my position and the college prefaces my account of the first year.

My Position

As with many pharmacy practice faculty, my responsibilities include teaching, research, clinical practice, and university service. My position at Oregon State University is tenure eligible; however, I have a two-year, fixed-term appointment (termed a "run-in period" in my contract) before my position is converted to tenure-track. This pushes back my university-level three-year and five-year reviews by two years. The option of a two-year run-in is offered to tenure-track pharmacy practice faculty at Oregon State University because of the time demands of developing a clinical practice. Ultimately, I think the two-year run-in period improves my likelihood of future success in establishing a research program because I do not have the dual pressures of clinical practice and research in the first and second years. The run-in period also gives me the opportunity to establish collaborative relationships and to identify and pilot areas of study.

I am fortunate that my contract describes many specific expectations for my position. For example, I need to plan to devote a minimum of 40% of my effort to scholarship, but a significant portion of my time in the first year may be devoted to establishing my responsibilities at the outpatient clinics. The areas receiving greatest emphasis for promotion and tenure will be teaching and research.

As a result of the restructuring of the College of Pharmacy that has occurred since a change of dean about nine months before I started my position, the Department of Pharmacy Practice has been granted permission by the university to hire non-tenure-track clinical faculty. The dean has offered practice faculty a one-time, six-month window of opportunity to move from tenure track to nontenure track. This has prompted me to take a hard look at my reasons for coming to Oregon State University in the first place.

When I was searching for my first academic position, I tried to learn about tenure–why tenure systems are used, why they are so controversial, what a person usually has to do to attain tenure, what happens if a person does not attain tenure, and so on. Armed with the vagaries that I was able to pick up about tenure, I then talked to pharmacists in tenure-track, non-tenure-track, and adjunct or volunteer positions to find out about the advantages and disadvantages of tenure-track, non-tenure-track, and volunteer affiliation. I learned that expectations for tenure track and nontenure track are very much dependent upon the university in question. Some universities have higher expectations for external funding and publication than others. Since faculty candidates seldom, if ever, are told the number of publications or dollars in external funding that are expected. I did Medline searches to find out how many and what types of articles senior faculty had published and guesstimated the amount and types of funding they brought in. I also talked to faculty members at various universities about the scholarly activities of their own faculty and those of their peers at other universities.

I also considered my training. Even though I did tailor my specialty residency to include more teaching and scholarly activity than most programs, many would argue that I am not qualified for a tenure-track position because I have not done a fellowship or do not have a Ph.D.

Finally, and most importantly, I considered my professional interests. Although I very much enjoy establishing new clinical services and helping patients, I think that I can have a greater impact on patient care and the profession of pharmacy by teaching students. I have known since graduating from high school that I wanted to teach at the university level. I like to write and want to contribute to the pharmacy and medical literature. I have another 35 or 40 years of work ahead of me. I do not want to restrict my career options. I want to grow and be challenged in my career.

One of the reasons that I first considered the position at Oregon State University was because it is tenure track. There are very few tenure-track positions available for ambulatory care faculty, probably because the time demands of a clinical practice make the development of a successful research program very difficult. Being given the opportunity to change from tenure track to nontenure track has prompted much research-related introspection and anxiety. I did not want to set myself up for failure, but I decided that it was worth the risk to remain in a tenure-track position. I am prepared, however, to look at my progress at my three-year review and make a tough decision about staying at Oregon State University, moving to a different school at a clinical track level, going to graduate school, or leaving academe entirely.

The College

The College of Pharmacy is in curricular transition. The last B.S. and post-B.S. Pharm.D. classes will graduate in 2001. The first entry-level Pharm.D. class will graduate in 2003. The first two years of the entry-level Pharm.D. program are taught on the main campus of Oregon State University in Corvallis. The second two years are taught on the campus of Oregon Health Sciences University (OHSU) in Portland. The Pharm.D. degree is jointly conferred by the two schools.

The Oregon State University and OHSU campuses are 75 miles apart. The majority of the pharmacy practice faculty members, including myself, are based in Portland. Because the College of Pharmacy's space on the OHSU campus is limited, I do not yet have office space with the rest of the pharmacy practice faculty. My office is in the Internal Medicine suite on the other side of the OHSU campus.

MY EXPERIENCES

In some respects, the first day on the job was like the first day of college classes as a student: the big, unfamiliar campus; the myriad of new faces; the buzz of productivity; and the sense of opportunity. It was a bit overwhelming. To help focus my thoughts and energies, one of the first things I did was write my mission statement.

Mission Statement 8/99

> As an educator, practitioner, and researcher, I am responsible for raising the level of pharmacy practice. I am responsible primarily for the training of pharmacy students. In providing clinical pharmacy services to the outpatient clinics, I am a role model to pharmacy students. Students' experiences will be practical and will prepare them to be practitioners in the "real world," wherever the target practice setting. I represent all of clinical pharmacy services to the providers in the clinic. My research questions, affirms, or refutes therapeutic modalities, teaching methods, or clinical pharmacy services in ambulatory care settings.

This vision provided direction and purpose to my daily activities during the first year. It helped me to stay focused on my responsibilities and goals. I think it might be a helpful exercise for other faculty members, whether they are new to academe or mid-career.

Teaching

My teaching responsibilities were limited during the first year, with the intention that I would have more time to devote to developing a clinical practice. Logistically, this has been possible because of the curriculum transition. During the first year, I was a preceptor for two students on ambulatory care rotations. I facilitated about a dozen small group sessions, and I attended the year-long weekly Pharm.D. seminar course. I did not teach any didactic courses.

I had a lot of autonomy in developing my ambulatory care rotation. The rotation I offer students is modeled after the practice environment of my second year of residency. The students conduct visits two or three half days per week with patients who are scheduled to see the clinical pharmacist at the Internal Medicine Clinic. These visits are typically for diabetes education or management, smoking cessation counseling, medication management or review, or hypertension management. The first day or two, I have the students observe visits that I conduct. Then I have them conduct the visit while I observe. Once I am comfortable with the students' skills and knowledge, the students conduct visits on their own and present patients to me for review before the patients leave. The students spend one half day per week at the Diabetes Center, seeing patients in conjunction with an endocrinologist. The students also rotate through a nurse-managed anticoagulation clinic for six half days. When they are not seeing patients, the students respond to drug information questions from the providers and work on various projects. The students also participate in a weekly journal club, present cases, and provide in-services at the clinics.

I prefer structure and objectives as a learner and find them even more important as a teacher since I am managing the students' learning experiences as well as my teaching, clinical, and research responsibilities. I compiled a student notebook that contains a description of the rotation, rotation objectives, expectations and assessment, information about key personnel with whom the students will interact, important numbers and resources, and key readings on ambulatory care practice. I developed a prerotation student assessment form specific for diabetes knowledge, skills, and attitudes that I use to tailor the rotation to the students' needs. I would like to expand the assessment to other disease states. At the beginning of the rotation, I give each student a calendar with clinic times, presentation dates, assignment deadlines, journal clubs, case conferences, preclinic conferences, and grand rounds. This organized approach keeps us on track and is appreciated by the students. At the American Association of Colleges of Pharmacy (AACP) 2000 Annual Meeting, I picked up some new ideas at the poster sessions that I am considering incorporating into the ambulatory care rotation. The dean strongly encouraged attendance at this meeting by all faculty members, and I am glad that I attended.

I enjoy teaching students on rotation. I definitely expend more energy and put in longer hours when students are with me. I invest a lot of time the first week, introducing students to the staff at the clinic and showing them where things are and how things work. I think the students do best when they feel that they are part of the team and understand their role. Despite my initial concerns that the students would take issue with my authority because of our similarity in age, the students have been respectfully receptive to my guidance and evaluation.

In my second year, I will be team teaching the ambulatory care rotation with two other ambulatory care faculty members. This should be beneficial for me because I will have a constant stream of students on rotation in the clinics for four half days per week, yet I will have blocks of time when I do not have patients scheduled and do not have students. I have been advised by many faculty members at Oregon State University and at other universities to protect my time for scholarly activity as much as possible.

Because the Pharm.D. entry-level curriculum is still in development, there are many uncertainties for me about didactic teaching responsibilities that will start when our first class reaches the third professional year, which will be my third year on faculty. As plans are finalized for the curriculum, I should have a clearer idea of my teaching load. The addition of didactic teaching to my schedule will provide a new set of challenges. Getting instructive feedback from senior faculty members on my lectures and handouts will be important to shaping my teaching style.

Coming into my position, I knew that I wanted to establish a specialty residency in ambulatory care. In my experience as a resident, many residency preceptors remarked that having a resident is one of the most rewarding aspects of their position. A good resident can also help increase practice and research productivity and assist with teaching responsibilities. The primary obstacle to directing a residency is usually obtaining and maintaining funding. I have been fortunate in that one of my colleagues at the College of Pharmacy offered to share the directorship of an ambulatory care/managed care specialty residency that has an established funding source. Our first resident will start as I go into my second year as a faculty member. I am looking forward to this teaching opportunity.

One of my other teaching-related goals, which has been encouraged by my department chair, is to obtain a joint faculty appointment at the level of Clinical Assistant Professor in the Department of Medicine at the School of Medicine. Dual appointments are looked upon favorably by the College of Pharmacy. The appointment in the Department of Medicine represents the teaching and support that I provide to medical students, medical residents, and faculty in the clinics. It is formal recognition of my contribution to interdisciplinary education and to scholarship in the Department of Medicine. While I cannot obtain reimbursement for the clinical services that I provide, I can contribute to the teaching mission through pharmacotherapy consultations and educational programs. In addition, much of my clinical research will be collaborative with primary faculty in the Department of Medicine. I requested the appointment through the clinic's medical director, who is also the Division Head of Internal Medicine in the Department of Medicine. She agreed that an appointment in the Department of Medicine was appropriate and provided the paperwork and a letter of recommendation.

Practice

The focus of my first year on faculty has been the development of an Internal Medicine Clinic practice site. I essentially started a new practice since a pharmacist had not practiced in the clinic for over three years, and in that time there had been a lot of turnover. Fortunately, the clinic's medical director strongly supports a multidisciplinary approach to patient care and learning. When I started, she outlined three areas with which the clinic needed help: medication refills and documentation, sample medications, and drug interactions. She also said, "Tell us and teach us what a clinical pharmacist can do because most of us do not know." She sent out an e-mail message to all of the clinic's faculty and staff announcing my arrival. I posted flyers and sent e-mail messages describing the clinical pharmacy services that I was offering, how to refer patients, and how providers could contact me for consults.

My services started out general–answering drug information questions, educating patients about their medications, and making pharmacotherapy recommendations. It took several months for me to understand the needs of the patient population and the providers. It took even longer to flesh out the needs of specific physicians. A few physicians immediately began to make referrals and to seek out drug information. Others were more tentative, only coming to me occasionally with questions. Over time, patterns of referrals and patients' needs became apparent. I am glad that I allowed the needs of the patients and the providers to shape the types of services that I provide, rather than going in with the intent of providing a particular service and hoping that there would be a need for it and that there would be support. If I had not taken the approach that I did, I would have lost several important areas of intervention, especially medication management in patients with complex medical illness and those with limited English-speaking abilities.

The first weeks and even couple of months of setting up clinical pharmacy services were tough. It seemed as though I was constantly explaining who I was, what I did, and why I was there. Even that was not easy: I was doing something that many of the staff had never heard of a pharmacist doing in the clinic, I was not employed by the clinic or the hospital, and I was not able to bill for my services. The staff would say, "Tell me again, why are you here?" I would remind them that I was there to establish clinical pharmacy services that support the experiential learning of pharmacy students as well as to provide the framework for my clinical research. I would go on to describe how it would be a win-win relationship for the clinic and the College of Pharmacy. The patients would get extra attention on their medication-related issues, the nurses and physicians would have a resource for medication questions, and pharmacy students would learn about the use of medicines in primary care. The look I read in most people's faces was, "Ok, whatever you say, let's see what you can do." Essentially, I would have to demonstrate my value.

As I was establishing my clinical practice, I pursued billing for services. I did this for two reasons. First, the care that I provide to patients is of value. I do not want to give away services. I did not think this would be a good precedent to set. Second, 100% of my salary comes from the College of Pharmacy. I do not think that the College of Pharmacy should pay me to provide care to patients, even if it is in the setting of teaching pharmacy students. After all, physician educators bill for patient visits on days that medical students are working with them. I reasoned that there are several ways to go about "recovering" the value of the clinical services that I provide. One way is through billing third-party insurance. Another is through contracting with the medical group or the capitated managed care plans. A third way is to apply for grants to develop and evaluate clinical pharmacy services and interdisciplinary educational programs. Although no one at the College of Pharmacy has formally said that recovering the value of the clinical services that I, or any of the other pharmacy practice faculty members, provide is an expectation, I do think that it is an avenue for bringing money back to the college that should be explored.

I began investigating reimbursement opportunities by making inquiries about whether OHSU and the medical practice were capable of or interested in billing for clinical pharmacy services. What I discovered was layer upon layer of administration and politics and very little reimbursement potential. It was a frustrating endeavor. There are a number of relationships through which I attempted to maneuver in my quest for billing: the complex relationship among the hospital, the clinics, and the physician groups; the delicate, although strengthening, relationship between the medical center's Department of Pharmacy and the College of Pharmacy; and the relationship between Oregon State University and OHSU. Probably the most important thing that I learned, though, was the importance of respecting the reporting structure that exists within large institutions and communicating as much as possible with the people in power.

Since third-party billing is not an option at present, I am hesitant to ask the medical group for a percentage of my salary. I cannot generate revenue from the overhead that I am currently using. I considered trying to set up contracts for service with the capitated managed care plans, but ultimately I decided that this was more than I wanted to get into. At this time, I will probably have more success pursuing grants to develop and evaluate clinical pharmacy services and interdisciplinary educational programs than going after third-party reimbursement or contracts with the medical group or managed care plans. And, hopefully, I will be able to turn the grant-funded projects into publications, making it a favorable scenario.

Beginning my career as the lone clinical pharmacy specialist in the outpatient clinics presented other challenges. I did not have anyone immediately available to critique my recommendations. I did not have anyone to explain personality idiosyncrasies or professional philosophies, such as, "Don't expect any referrals from Dr. So-and-So because she likes to manage her patients herself." Most of my venting was done long distance via e-mail or phone with one of my residency preceptors. I was reluctant to go to the other ambulatory care faculty members at my college because I did not want their primary impression of me to be that I was struggling or that I was a complainer. I was just hitting a few bumps in the road.

Midway through my first year, I came upon an unexpected opportunity. I was offered the responsibilities of a clerkship site of a preceptor who was leaving the College of Pharmacy. I think I got every new clinical faculty member's dream: I inherited an established relationship with a physician who is a former clinical pharmacist, a great teacher for pharmacy students, a role model for patient teaching, a clinical researcher, and a specialty practitioner in one of my areas of interest. This relationship has been vital to the development of my clinical and research network at OHSU.

Perhaps I have taken on more projects and responsibilities in my clinical practice than a seasoned faculty member would. Many of the opportunities which on the surface looked like "time drainers" have actually been extremely important to the growth of my practice and to the support of my research. For example, one of the services that I provide for the Internal Medicine Clinic is simply "medication management," which includes educating patients about their medications, making medication lists, and filling medication boxes. Through this service, I discovered a patient population that appears to be underserved by the current system of providing pharmaceutical care. I am now undertaking a major research initiative to study medication use in non-English-speaking patients.

Professional credentialing and involvement in the American College of Clinical Pharmacy (ACCP) Ambulatory Care Practice and Research Network (PRN) have also been important aspects of my first year. I took the Board Certified Pharmacotherapy Specialists (BCPS) examination and the Certified Diabetes Educator (CDE) examination in my third month as a faculty member. At that time the information was fresh. I was motivated, and my teaching responsibilities were minimal. I am glad that I pursued these credentials when I did. It was an important accomplishment to pass the BCPS exam because it seems to have become a rite of passage among new clinical pharmacy specialists, especially those who are faculty members. The CDE credential has been important for my acceptance among other diabetes educators and appears to have improved the confidence of some physicians in my abilities as a diabetes educator. The ACCP Ambulatory Care Practice and Research Network listserv and networking sessions have been useful resources in developing my practice.

Now that I am established in the internal medicine and specialty practices, my next step is to redefine my clinical services such that there is a stronger overlap with my research efforts. One way that I will do this is by delegating some clinical responsibilities to my resident. Another way will be to focus my energies in areas where there is external funding or where there is potential for external funding. And, of course, one of the most important and probably most challenging ways to establish a stronger overlap between my clinical services and my research efforts will be to begin to say "no" and be more selective in my activities.

Research

One reason I took this position is that it offers me the opportunity to put a substantial amount of time into scholarly activity. This is a challenge for me because the focus of my training was in practice and not research. In my first year as a faculty member, my three research-related objectives have been to establish relationships that will foster collaborative research, to participate in workshops and seminars that will improve my research skills, and to identify research support services and granting agencies.

I have found the physicians with whom I work in the clinic to be supportive of my research ideas. A couple of the physicians who are more research intensive regularly bring ideas to me now. I have the sense that I am building momentum with other providers as they become aware of my interest in and ability to contribute to scholarly activities. I am making inroads at establishing relationships with pharmacy faculty and area pharmacists. Two of the pharmacy faculty members are especially interested in collaborative research, and we are embarking on several projects. One of the more senior faculty members, in particular, has provided me with opportunities to tap into his population-based approach to research through collaboration with a managed care organization. My vision is that this type of initial collaborative research will continue to grow to the extent that I will be able to sustain an independent research program.

I attended several research skill development programs this year. In addition to the university's standard introduction to the research office and the required human subjects training, I attended the American Association of Colleges of Pharmacy (AACP)/American College of Clinical Pharmacists (ACCP) Grant Writing Seminar, the ACCP Annual Meeting research-track presentations, and an Oregon State University proposal-writing workshop. I am also taking an on-line grant-writing course. I keep a file of grant opportunities and a calendar of the deadlines. Many of the programs I attended recommended setting aside an hour each day to write. I am determined to do this on a regular basis in my second year as a faculty member.

When I started at Oregon State University, I knew there were resources available to support new faculty research; I just was not sure how to get connected. Information about research support services, such as statistical services and survey development, has been trickling in via e-mail, casual conversations, and university programming. I have been slowly discovering training and development opportunities at the OHSU

General Clinical Research Center. I have been building a file of these research support services. This is something that would have been helpful to have when I started. Although many of the faculty members have reassured me that they can provide assistance with navigating proposals and budgets between both Oregon State University and OHSU, these are still two of the more elusive aspects of the research process for me.

Overall, I am excited to begin studying a few of the many therapeutic, teaching, and clinical service questions with which I seem to be deluged. I keep a file of ideas for research projects and review articles; it is bulging. I also have a file in my Palm Pilot for ideas that occur to me outside the office. I have a quotation from Thomas Edison on my office bulletin board that says, "If we all did the things we are capable of doing, we would literally astound ourselves." Prioritizing and narrowing my focus are my current challenges in the area of research.

Service

I serve on two College of Pharmacy search committees and on the extended-education committee. I have learned a lot about the college and faculty members' interests by working on the search committees. It has been a good experience. My time commitment to these committees has been modest, which I think is appropriate for a new faculty member.

At OHSU, I serve on three committees: the Internal Medicine Clinic Care Management Team, the Internal Medicine Leadership Team, and the Diabetes Task Force. My participation on these committees has been important to my success at developing clinical services and establishing collaborative relationships. To what extent this service counts toward promotion and tenure, I will need to clarify before my tenure clock starts.

My service within the profession includes participating on the board of one pharmacy organization and on a committee of another. I would like to advise a student organization once we have the entry-level Pharm.D. students in Portland. I benefited a great deal from organizational involvement as a student, so I would like to foster professionalism and leadership skills in our students through professional organizations as an advisor.

Collegiality

The majority of my time has been spent in my office at the clinic and in the clinic itself. This has enabled me to develop strong collegial relationships with the medical faculty and staff. However, I feel somewhat removed from the pharmacy practice faculty because my office is on the other side of campus. Office space at the OHSU campus is sparse. It is not uncommon for new practice faculty to only have offices or cubbyholes at their practice sites. I "visit" the college to check my mail, to attend meetings, and, occasionally, to teach. I do not know the pharmacy faculty as well as I would like. We have only had three "monthly" departmental meetings during the first year. The infrequent meetings, along with not having an office with the rest of the faculty, have been barriers to my acclimation to the faculty and my sense of teamwork. Although I have been assured that we will have more departmental meetings in the coming year, I need to make a better effort at becoming part of the team.

Three new faculty members, including myself, started around the same time. One of the more senior faculty members from the college had a welcoming party for us. This was a great way to get to know everyone on a more personal basis. Since then, we have met as a faculty three more times on a purely social basis. There are a couple of faculty members with whom I get together on a regular basis outside of work. These friendships have provided good escapes from the stresses and long hours of work.

I think it is difficult for most of our practice faculty to establish and maintain productive relationships with the basic science faculty and vice versa because we are on different campuses. The relationship that the practice faculty has with the basic science faculty is collegial. I get the sense that both groups would like more interaction. At this time, I am satisfied with the relationship. I feel there are several basic science faculty members I could approach to review grant proposals or to ask advice about promotion and tenure. The full faculty has met twice in the first year for meetings. We interacted on a more social basis at the dean's holiday party and at the graduate retreat, where faculty members come together to hear presentations by the graduate students and Pharm.D. candidates.

Mentorship

A mentor is someone who guides and facilitates. A mentor gives you a map, points out ruts in the roads, and lets you go, go, go. I have a mentor from my second residency. She has been an incredibly important source of guidance, comfort, and encouragement during this first year. I do not have a formal mentor at Oregon State University, yet. There is no formal mentoring program, although there are plans for one. I would like to have a formal mentoring program in place. Several faculty members have provided important "curbside" mentoring, such as inquiring how I am doing in developing clinical services, encouraging me not to get too wrapped up in providing clinical service, giving advice on record keeping for my dossier, and offering to review manuscripts and proposals.

The person who models teaching and leadership for me most right now is the director of the Internal Medicine Clinic. I like her listening and problem-solving styles and the way she interacts with students, residents, and faculty. She is an enabler. Her interest is in education, and her drive is to study educational processes and outcomes. I have benefited greatly from the teaching in-services that are presented at the monthly section meeting of Internal Medicine, which she chairs. She has many qualities that I try to emulate.

University Interface

Although my office is not physically located on the Oregon State University campus, I am as connected as I want to be. I receive e-mail about goings-on. I receive the campus paper and the College of Pharmacy newsletter. The interface with which I am more concerned is OHSU. Many of the practice faculty teach, provide service, do research, use library resources, and rely on the network support services of OHSU, but the College of Pharmacy is not formally recognized as an entity of OHSU. A business plan between the College of Pharmacy and OHSU is under development. The business plan is essential for having facilities to train our students in the classroom and in practice. I think that the business plan is also important from the perspective of a researcher whose primary study site is at one university and promotion and tenure system is at the other.

GENERAL

The essence of my orientation as a new faculty member was really just all of the experiences that I brought with me. It has taken patience and persistence to make it through the first year. Much of the attractiveness of being a faculty member is the autonomy; however, it has been difficult for me to appreciate the autonomy in the first year. The autonomy has seemed more like "do it yourself" rather than a stimulus for creativity. I cannot deny that it was a stressful year.

A friend who is considering a career in academe recently commented, "It seems like people in faculty positions are constantly balancing a huge number of projects and still have more ideas they want to study than they will ever have time for." There is a certain amount of anxiety that goes along with balancing 10 to 20 projects at various stages of completion. It is truly amazing that anything ever gets done. On top of that, I am trying to find a balance between work and everything else. I suspect, however, that I will be grappling with the balances of work and free time/family time throughout my career.

One of the more important reasons that I accepted this position at Oregon State University is that it puts me closer to family. My only sibling and his wife are within driving distance, which makes it easier for us to visit as a family when my parents fly out from the Midwest. The Northwest is an appealing place to live. Portland is a metropolitan area with a small-town feel. I do miss the sun sometimes, but the lush green of the trees and the mountains help to make up for it. I am glad to be part of a community again after being in two different cities during my residencies. It is beginning to feel like home.

Two years of hindsight is not enough to enable me to read into a lot of the naivety, successes, and misadventures that I have described. It has been a helpful exercise to think through it and write about it. I have accomplished more than I realized, and I had more structure and purpose going about my accomplishments than I thought. I also identified areas that I want to improve. I hope this description provides useful insight to current and future new faculty, senior colleagues, and pharmacy administrators.

New Challenges, New Opportunities: Perspective of a New Faculty Member

Scott K. Stolte

As I begin to write, it is difficult for me to believe that I have been a faculty member for two years. It seems only a short time ago that I walked through the doors of the school wondering where this road I had chosen would lead me. I would not say that the road has always been a smooth one, nor has it always been bumpy. It has certainly not been what I expected at times, and it has surpassed my expectations at other times. I can say with certainty that the road, for me, has been the right one.

I chose a career in academe primarily because I felt that I wanted to teach. I say I felt I wanted to teach because I had limited experience in teaching prior to accepting my position at Shenandoah University. I simply knew it was what I wanted to do. My own educational experience at Purdue University was excellent, and I developed a strong respect and admiration for many of my instructors and professors there. I saw their commitment to making us good students; but, more than that, I felt they wanted to make us outstanding pharmacists and future colleagues. My desire was to bring this same dedication to another group of future pharmacists. The opportunities I had to teach pharmacy students as a part of my residency experience were very rewarding and were the part of the residency I most enjoyed. Also, during my resi-

---

Scott K. Stolte, Pharm.D., formerly Assistant Professor of Pharmacy Practice at Shenandoah University, is now in Biopharmaceutical Medical Affairs at Novo Nordisk Pharmaceuticals, Inc., 100 College Road West, Princeton, NJ 08540.

[Haworth co-indexing entry note]: "New Challenges, New Opportunities: Perspective of a New Faculty Member." Stolte, Scott K. Co-published simultaneously in *Journal of Pharmacy Teaching* (Pharmaceutical Products Press, an imprint of The Haworth Press, Inc.) Vol. 9, No. 1, 2002, pp. 35-45; and: *Handbook for Pharmacy Educators: Getting Adjusted As a New Pharmacy Faculty Member* (ed: Shane P. Desselle and Dana P. Hammer) Pharmaceutical Products Press, an imprint of The Haworth Press, Inc., 2002, pp. 35-45. Single or multiple copies of this article are available for a fee from The Haworth Document Delivery Service [1-800-HAWORTH, 9:00 a.m. - 5:00 p.m. (EST). E-mail address: getinfo@haworthpressinc.com].

© 2002 by The Haworth Press, Inc. All rights reserved.

dency, I had the opportunity to speak and give presentations at various local, state, and national events. The participants in these programs often told me that I was among the best lecturers they had experienced. People still tell me that. I am not certain what it is about my personality or my lecture style that others enjoy. It may be that I care about the content I am teaching because I feel it is essential to being a good pharmacist, but probably more importantly, I care about the students and participants I am teaching.

So, how did I choose to come to Shenandoah University? The university is located in Winchester, Virginia, which is a small town in the beautiful Shenandoah Valley of northern Virginia. I grew up approximately one hour north of the school in south central Pennsylvania. When I first started looking at faculty positions, I wanted to look in an area of the country where I had never lived. I did not want to be limited by geographical constraints. However, geography played a big part in my choosing Shenandoah over a number of other positions. Right about the time I began my search for faculty positions, my stepfather was diagnosed with renal cell carcinoma. It was important to me that I was close by to spend time with him and support my mother and younger brother during this very difficult period.

I did not expect there to be much of an adjustment period because I had been in this area of the country for most of my life, but there certainly was. The biggest adjustment was moving from a university of approximately 40,000 students to one with just a few thousand. I missed, and still miss, the home football Saturdays at Ross-Ade stadium, the basketball games at Mackey Arena, the Co-Rec gymnasium complex where I exercised with friends, the constant buzz of activity that exists at large universities, and the many choices available when you are trying to find something to do in the evening and on weekends. Winchester and Shenandoah University do not offer these options, but there are advantages to small schools also. I will expound on these advantages later. Just to let you know, Shenandoah has recently fielded a football team. This does not exactly make up for all of the activities I miss, but it is an initial step in the right direction.

In addition to everything that I was considering, I had to consider the needs of my wife. Like me, she grew up in south central Pennsylvania, so she was looking forward to being close to her family again. However, she had also established herself in Indiana. She is an elementary teacher and was teaching at a school located in a rural town just outside of Lafayette. She really enjoyed the children and the parents she worked with there. If any of you have experience or spouses with experience in finding an elementary teaching position, you know it is no easy task. At the time we moved, she had applied for teaching positions in Winchester and the surrounding areas but had not received any interview invitations or offers. I suppose that any time you leave an area you make sacrifices; so, based on all the considerations, we felt that it was the best decision for us at that time. The people I had met at the interview at Shenandoah were great, and I knew that I would be able to start teaching right away. These were the aspects I focused on as we packed our bags and moved from Indiana to Virginia.

Teaching is basically all I knew academe to be when I started because it was all I had ever seen. As a student and resident, I did not have the opportunity to witness what goes on behind the scenes. I walked into my office on the first day of my new job and started to write the lectures I would be delivering in the first couple weeks of the fall semester. I remember thinking to myself that this was a pretty good deal—writing lectures and teaching them to students. What was I going to do with all the spare time? I have always enjoyed autonomy because I usually have no trouble finding productive ways to keep myself busy. In fact, this was one consideration in choosing a smaller, teaching-focused school. I felt I would have more opportunity to determine for myself what was important. In general, I still believe this is true and is something worth considering when searching for the school with the best fit. Writing those initial lectures, I had no idea that there is so much involved in being a faculty member. It did not take me long to realize that teaching is only one component of the job. It will always be the most important component to me, but there is also research, school and university service, developing relationships with other faculty members, and student advising and mentoring. I soon found that the free time had disappeared (partly because of my inherent inability to say no to opportunities and challenges) and that the task became balancing all the demands for time and energy that are placed on a faculty member. I hope my description of the different aspects of my position will allow new faculty members to achieve the balance that I am still looking for. In addition, I hope it allows senior faculty and administrators to identify areas where they can provide support for new faculty.

At Shenandoah, the faculty members teach a wide array of courses reflecting their vast diversity of expertise. There is a strong emphasis on quality teaching at the school and the university. This is evidenced by the fact that there are numerous awards at both levels for quality teaching (School Teacher of the Year, University Student Government citations, etc.) and relatively few research-based rewards. Also, a good teaching record as defined by peer and student evaluation is required for promotion at the university. I have heard from some of my new faculty colleagues across the country that they were not required to teach didactic lectures during their first semester or even first year in their position. That was not the case for me. I arrived at the school on July 20, 1998, with the expectation that I would be delivering 6 hours of lectures for the gastrointestinal module in 1 month.

Preparing lectures for the classroom at Shenandoah is slightly different than what is required at most schools. All of our course materials, including handouts and slides, are posted on the World Wide Web for the students to access. This is convenient for the students and faculty, but it does require some additional preparation, including entering your lectures into defined web-based templates and handling web copyright issues. When I started, I felt like I was technologically savvy. I soon realized that there is a big difference between word processing and web authoring.

Most often, I teach in the integrated care sequence of courses. This is similar to the traditional therapeutics courses offered at most schools, except that pharmacology and medicinal chemistry are integrated with pharmacotherapeutics into one course. Integrated care (ICARE) is broken down by disease states or organ systems into 11 smaller courses (e.g., neurosensory, infectious disease). I teach approximately 20 to 30 classroom hours each semester in these courses. In addition, I lecture in some of the Pharmacy Administration courses and facilitate one or two sections of the ICARE laboratory and two of our Nontraditional Doctor of Pharmacy teams. All of this adds up to approximately 8 to 10 hours per week of actual classroom time.

Until recently, I was responsible for serving as a liaison between all of the school's community pharmacy rotation sites and preceptors and the Chair of the Department of Pharmacy Practice. Recently, I was asked to begin precepting students in a community clinical rotation at a Rite Aid pharmacy close to the school. I will be assigned two students per six-week rotation block. I will work with the students to manage patients with a number of primary care disease states such as asthma and diabetes. Any faculty member who has ever precepted students knows that the majority of the time spent at the practice site with students present is spent teaching in some form. I estimate I will spend approximately two days per week with the students at the rotation site.

This probably sounds like quite a bit of time spent teaching, but it is just the right amount for me. It allows the students to get to know my teaching style and my expectations while allowing me to get to know them in a didactic as well as experiential setting. My style of teaching in the classroom and in the practice setting has been described by many students as "demanding but fair." In general, I agree with this assessment. I try to present the most current information in a way that is interesting and stimulating. I put quite a bit of time and energy into my didactic and experiential teaching. In return, I expect the students to put at least the same amount of effort into learning the material and applying it.

I think my teaching philosophy is well exemplified in a quotation I was given that now permanently resides above my computer monitor. It is from Ronda Beamon and reads, "Teaching is about igniting that flame, that desire of students to learn for themselves, not you. To do this work of learning because it means something in their life, not yours." I realize that many will feel this is idealistic for today's student. I have not found this to be the case. I am careful to explain to the students my expectations of them and what their expectations of me should be. By setting the ground rules up front, a tremendous amount of respect between us is established. For the most part, this respect is reflected in the performance of the student. This is not to say that every student in every class or every rotation will perform up to your expectations because that is certainly not the case. But, most give me their best effort because they realize they are receiving my best, and I am willing to accept that.

There are a few pointers I can provide from my personal experience to help anyone who is anxious about their initial classroom experiences. First, organization is infinitely more important than quantity. Believe it or not, there is no student who is going to learn everything there is to know about every topic. In organizing your lectures, present the must-know elements in such a way that students realize the importance of those points. This is probably the biggest single change I have implemented in my first few years of teaching. I try to take a few key points or ideas, teach them until I am sure the students understand them, and then fill in the remaining time with other, less essential, but still important content.

This brings me to another aspect of teaching that I was not particularly prepared for as a new faculty member: grading. I strongly feel that this is an area of academics that does not receive nearly enough attention. As a pharmacy student, I was keenly aware of my grades, and this focus on grades has not changed in the few years that I have been out of pharmacy school. However, one thing that is different in just those few years is the expectations of the students. This difference in expectation may be explained by a difference in academic settings or the students themselves, but it has become apparent that average is no longer acceptable to the students. When I was in school, it was expected that some students would receive *A* grades, some would receive *F* grades, and most would receive grades somewhere in between. The current perception is that a *C* grade is not acceptable. In speaking with colleagues around the country, I have found that this perception is not unique to Shenandoah. I do not believe in and do not abide by this philosophy. The definition of a *C* grade is and has always been average. I explain to my students that being average in a classroom of very intelligent people taking professional-level courses is not something of which to be ashamed. In fact, it is something of which they should be proud. Of course, not every student buys into this wisdom, but by explaining this to the students, I have greatly decreased the number of complaints I receive at the end of a course. I find no joy at all in issuing a sub-par grade to a student. However, we are teaching students who will be health professionals. We are training students who are going to be taking care of our friends, spouses, parents, and children. In my opinion, we have a duty to ensure that these students are capable and competent.

I feel peer mentoring and evaluation are very important to optimal performance as a faculty member. In my postgraduate training, I received excellent mentoring from my residency advisors. I owe much of my desire to be a dedicated pharmacist and educator to them. I consider myself a self-starter, and I did not require frequent guidance or encouragement. However, it was comforting to know that my mentors were there if I needed them. One of my mentors, who also served as my residency director, performed regular periodic evaluations of my performance. I was also evaluated by the students I precepted. At Shenandoah, I continue to be evaluated by students in the classroom, but we have no formal mentoring system or peer evaluation system in place. Although I feel student evaluation is important, I do not think it should be the only method used for evaluation. In general, my experience has been that students tend to penalize demanding instructors or those who grade stringently. Instructors should not be punished for the demands that they place on students. In addition to formal peer evaluation, I think all schools should have a formal mentoring program, with a senior faculty member assigned as a mentor to provide guidance. Most new faculty members have limited experience in the classroom, and it would be helpful to receive tips from someone seasoned in classroom teaching. The mentor could serve as a research mentor for the junior faculty member as well.

Overall, teaching was the reason that I chose a career in academe, and it is the reason I will stay for some time. Yes, you have issues that develop with students. Sometimes you even have conflicts with other faculty. But, when you are standing in front of the class teaching a particularly difficult topic and you see on the students' faces that they understand–you see that "flame of learning"–it is all worthwhile.

I really did not have a good understanding of what was meant by "service" until I started at the school. As most of you know, service is work that a faculty member performs for the benefit of the school, university, profession of pharmacy, or community. These activities contribute to the professional growth of faculty members and students. At Shenandoah, we have a relatively small faculty, so each new faculty member usually has the opportunity to serve on a committee at the school level if he or she so desires. Since standing committees for the school and university for upcoming academic years are formed in the previous May, new faculty members may not get to serve on these committees, but there are many ad hoc and search committees formed throughout the year on which a new faculty member can serve. Service is a necessary component of productivity and is considered when one is evaluated for promotion at the school. However, there are no service-based rewards at the school level and very few at the university level. Over the past two years, I have been involved with the Faculty Affairs Committee, the Student-Faculty Liaison Committee, the Nontraditional Doctor of Pharmacy Experiential Committee, and a number of ad hoc and search committees.

The work of the Faculty Affairs Committee at Shenandoah has been fairly intensive because the school is relatively new and is still developing many of the policies and procedures that established schools have had more time to develop. This committee represents the entire faculty for the school and advocates for faculty welfare. Activities of this committee have included the development of promotion criteria for the school, the implementation of experiential evaluation forms for our students on rotation, and the revision and implementation of classroom evaluation forms that are used by the students to evaluate the faculty of the school. Many other issues are brought to the committee by the faculty.

The Student-Faculty Liaison Committee addresses unique and challenging situations. The charge of this committee is to hear cases on student conduct upon complaint of faculty or others. Although the work of this committee is not as intensive as that of the Faculty Affairs Committee, it is difficult because it often involves levying sanctions upon students in the school. Although committee work in general can be time consuming and demanding on a professional and personal level, I enjoy it because it gives me the opportunity to work side by side with the other faculty of the school. My fellow faculty members were the main reason I chose to come to Shenandoah University.

The collegiality among the faculty at Shenandoah has been everything I could ask for and more. When I accepted the position, I was concerned about developing relationships with my colleagues. Everyone seemed personable at the interview, but I did not really know anyone. It was incredibly helpful to be starting with other new faculty in my department. I realize not everyone will have this luxury when starting an academic position, but it was nice for all of us to get our feet wet together.

Approximately one month after I arrived at the school, a two-day faculty/staff retreat was held away from the school. This went a long way toward building a collegial climate among faculty and staff. In fact, if there is one recommendation I would make to deans or department chairs looking to enhance relationships among faculty, it is to have an overnight retreat away from campus. The year after that initial retreat, we had a two-day retreat at the school, and it did not seem to establish the fellowship that the gathering away from campus did.

In addition to having good social relationships with my fellow faculty members, we have mutually beneficial professional relationships as well. I am often called on to do a lecture in another faculty member's course if the topic is within my areas of expertise. Likewise, I feel comfortable asking other faculty members to provide expertise in my courses. Much of the research currently being conducted at the school is in conjunction with other faculty members, both within the same department and among other departments. There is seldom a competitive nature to these projects, and they end up being great learning experiences for all involved.

This brings me to my research. Like many clinical practitioners finishing a practice residency, this is the part of this position I feared most. Shenandoah is a non-tenure-track university, but research is still required for promotion. From what I have seen, it is similar to a number of the pharmacy schools located at smaller private colleges and universities. In general, these schools tend to focus on service and teaching for promotion more and focus on research less. At first, this made me comfortable. However, after some thought, I realized that the chances of spending my entire career at Shenandoah were very slim. It is not that I do not like being here, but people tend to move on. I needed to think about what would be required of faculty in my position at other schools that have a greater emphasis on research. What if I someday wanted to be hired and promoted at one of these schools? I encourage all new faculty members to think about this possibility as they develop a research plan, especially if they are at an institution that does not place a heavy emphasis on research. Start thinking about a research agenda soon after you start your new faculty career.

It did not take me long to realize that the time I would be able to dedicate to research would be an important consideration. When compared with the amount of time spent in the classroom, the extra time spent with students outside the classroom, and the time spent in school and university service, research time is fairly limited. I decided to focus my research in the area of practice-based research. This worked out well for me initially for a number of reasons. First, this is the only type of research I had ever conducted. Second, I would be able to use the students on rotation and the pharmacists I worked with at the practice sites to help conduct the research. Finally, and most importantly to me at the time, there was and still is very little clinical research in the area of community pharmacy. I had met many community pharmacists who were delivering innovative and highly successful care to patients, but few of them had the time and/or the desire to publish what they were doing. I decided to focus my research efforts on disease management programs conducted in community pharmacies.

To get started with this effort, I developed an asthma disease management program designed to be delivered to patients in community pharmacies and ambulatory care clinics. I identified Kroger as a company that wanted to implement the program in its pharmacies. Kroger is a large grocery store chain with community pharmacies located within many of its stores. I oriented its pharmacists to the program in a two-day continuing education session at the company's regional headquarters. At approximately the same time, I oriented our students who had been assigned to do their community clinical rotations at Kroger to the program. The primary objective of the program was to show improvement in clinical and humanistic outcomes in patients being managed by the pharmacists and students. Patient results are still being collected and tabulated at this time, but preliminary results look positive.

Not long after this program was initiated, a colleague from Shenandoah and a pharmacy resident joined me to author a grant proposal for a project that would demonstrate the effectiveness of diabetes disease management in an independent community pharmacy. Again, the objective was to improve clinical and humanistic outcomes in the patients. We submitted a grant proposal to the Institute for the Advancement of Community Pharmacy for the project early this year. Recently, we received the news that the grant had been funded, and the project will be initiated soon.

In addition to practice-based research, I have had the opportunity to engage in research on educational strategies as well. I worked with two other faculty colleagues at the school in an effort to determine if preadmission indicators such as quantitative PCAT scores, performance on a basic math skills assessment test, demographic, and scholastic information were useful as a gauge of basic math skills for entering Doctor of Pharmacy candidates. This investigation was submitted for publication. Also, together with three other faculty members at the school, I submitted an article discussing how technological advances such as the Internet and synchronous chat have influenced pharmacy education. I have found that much of my writing takes place during semester breaks when there are few or no students at the school.

Probably the greatest surprise I have had in my current position to this point is that I really enjoy the research and writing I have done. As my practice site becomes more established and the developmental work of a new school begins to settle down, I look forward to spending more time in these endeavors. For now, I feel that the time that I have had to devote to this work has not been optimal, but I have been able to get some work done. I have found my department chair and the other administrators at the school to be extremely supportive of my research ideas. They have always encouraged me to pursue my interests. Keep in mind that most of the research I have completed does not require the purchase of expensive equipment and requires very little overhead to conduct. I cannot speculate on how these factors would affect the support I currently receive from the school's administration.

As you can see from my brief descriptions, the environment for collaboration among faculty members at the school is very good. We call on one another to contribute in areas of an individual strength, similarly to the way we call on one another to contribute in the classroom. As mentioned earlier, there is little feeling of competition. We tend to abide by the rule that the person who does the most work for a project is the first listed author, and the person who does the least amount of work is the author listed last. Due to the size and focus of the school and the university, I do not have graduate students to contribute to my research or writing. This somewhat limits the number of projects I can be involved in at any given time, but it allows me to completely focus my efforts in areas that are most interesting to me.

One resource that remains underutilized at this time is collaborative research with other health professions at the university. Shenandoah University has schools of nursing, physical therapy, occupational therapy, respiratory therapy, and a physician's assistant program. There are many opportunities for the pharmacy faculty to engage in interdepartmental research, and I encourage all who read this article to investigate similar opportunities at their schools. Research is the aspect of my position that I feared most when I accepted my position, but it is an aspect that I have found extremely rewarding and exciting. I encourage new faculty to start their research programs in areas that interest them and expand interests from that point. Also, do not hesitate to ask other faculty members for help if it is an area within their expertise. By engaging in collaborative research, I have accomplished much more than I would have if I had tried to conduct research all on my own.

Although some of my reflections on the first two years as a faculty member are unique, many of the fears and triumphs I have experienced are similar to those of my colleagues across the country. No, not everyone has had to address the sadness of losing a loved one or the anticipation and joy associated with a spouse starting a new career (second-grade teacher in Winchester) or the birth of a son (Daniel 7/18/99), but we all started with the ambiguity associated with not being sure what we were supposed to be doing because we were new at the position. Now, most of us have the feeling of not being sure what to do now because there is not enough time in the day. I am looking forward to spending more time in academe. I find great satisfaction in pursuing a career where I am continually challenged to learn new information and generate new ideas, develop expertise in these areas, and pass that expertise on to the students I teach. I was especially proud in May 1999 when the first group of pharmacy graduates in the history of Shenandoah University crossed the stage. As they were receiving their diplomas, I found myself asking whether I had given my best for these students. Were they, in fact, the health care providers I wanted taking care of my family and friends? I am proud of the answer that I was able to give, and I look forward to answering that question affirmatively for many years to come.

And You Think Your Job Stinks? Think Again: Every Cloud Does Have a Silver Lining

Gireesh V. Gupchup

Teaching is not a lost art, but the regard for it is a lost tradition.

– *Jacques Barzun*

A poor surgeon hurts 1 person at a time. A poor teacher hurts 130.

– *Ernest Boyer*

IN THE BEGINNING

The job seemed perfect. I would join a division that included an internationally renowned pharmacy administration faculty member, another junior faculty member would join soon, and an endowed chair would follow. Additionally, the college had a graduate program that included both M.S. and Ph.D. degrees. There seemed to be several research op-

---

Gireesh V. Gupchup, Ph.D., is Assistant Professor of Pharmacy, Concentration Chair for the Pharmacy Administration Graduate Program, and Director of the New Mexico Medicaid Retrospective Drug Utilization Review Program, College of Pharmacy, Health Sciences Center, University of New Mexico, Albuquerque, NM 87131 (E-mail: gupchup@unm.edu).

[Haworth co-indexing entry note]: "And You Think Your Job Stinks? Think Again: Every Cloud Does Have a Silver Lining." Gupchup, Gireesh V. Co-published simultaneously in *Journal of Pharmacy Teaching* (Pharmaceutical Products Press, an imprint of The Haworth Press, Inc.) Vol. 9, No. 1, 2002, pp. 47-59; and: *Handbook for Pharmacy Educators: Getting Adjusted As a New Pharmacy Faculty Member* (ed: Shane P. Desselle and Dana P. Hammer) Pharmaceutical Products Press, an imprint of The Haworth Press, Inc., 2002, pp. 47-59. Single or multiple copies of this article are available for a fee from The Haworth Document Delivery Service [1-800-HAWORTH, 9:00 a.m. - 5:00 p.m. (EST). E-mail address: getinfo@haworthpressinc.com].

© 2002 by The Haworth Press, Inc. All rights reserved.

portunities with faculty who were willing to help mentor me. The city's year-round recreational activities, pleasant climate, cultural diversity, and geographic beauty were big pluses. Although I had several interviews pending, I could not refuse the job.

During my first day on the job, things changed. I found out that the senior faculty member had retired, the junior faculty member who was expected to join soon would not do so for at least two years, and the possibility of obtaining an endowed chair was not as promising as it seemed when I interviewed for the job. Essentially, I was the only pharmacy administration faculty member, and I had to coordinate four courses that started in two weeks! Also, I was told that I would have to chair the graduate program, for which I quickly learned we had little financial support from the college. Was it already time to throw in the towel?

I could have, but I didn't, partly because it was difficult to move my family again and partly because I remembered that my mother always said, "Everything happens for the better." Most importantly, I treated the situation as an opportunity. It was a rare situation in which few pharmacy faculty members would find themselves. That is what makes a narrative of my experiences unique.

From the perspective of the college, it was not possible to predict the retirement of the internationally renowned faculty member. With regard to the hiring of a junior faculty member and the endowed chair, it was probably partly my fault for not asking the correct questions. I also believe that a college has a responsibility to clarify what hurdles a new faculty member may have to clear after joining. In retrospect, I should have asked specific questions about the time frame in which these positions would be filled. In my excitement to join what I believed was a "perfect position," I didn't analyze the situation well enough. My advice to budding faculty members would be to talk with experienced faculty members at their institution about the *realistic* demands that a particular position may entail once you have visited a prospective college. For example, it sounds great that one would have an opportunity to guide graduate students. However, the amount of effort required to guide graduate students may not be apparent to a fresh Ph.D. graduate, even if the work proves very rewarding.

In the remainder of this article, I will describe how I handled the challenges in research, teaching, service, mentoring, and interaction with college and university-wide faculty that have presented themselves during my four years in New Mexico. I hope the account of both my successful experiences and, more importantly, my mistakes will help junior faculty in their future careers and help experienced faculty understand current challenges faced by new faculty.

RESEARCH

When I joined the University of New Mexico, I was informed that we were a Carnegie Research I University. At that time it didn't mean much to me. I learned during my first year on the job that this meant that our university was among the top extramurally funded institutions in the U.S. Although I was informed during my interview that I was required to get grants and publish papers regularly, only when I joined the faculty did I realize that this was no easy task. I was always interested in research, and that helped me. However, it took at least three years for me to figure out what I wanted to focus on in terms of research.

What helped me early on in my research endeavors was that one of my former professors, Dr. Mike Rupp, introduced me to pharmacists at the Indian Health Service (IHS) Hospital in Albuquerque. They were getting ready to implement a pharmaceutical care plan for asthma patients. During discussions with the IHS pharmacists, it was determined that in order for us to document the outcomes of patients resulting from the implementation of pharmaceutical care plans, we needed to develop a questionnaire specifically for measuring quality-of-life for asthma patients. This project landed me my first grant during my first semester at New Mexico. The culturally-specific nature of this health-related quality of life (HRQOL) questionnaire allowed me to make several contacts with researchers who have similar interests both within and outside the university.

Obtaining a grant for the above-mentioned project was not easy. Before I finally received a grant from the University Research Allocations Committee, I was told by two external agencies that encouraged research in minority populations that I was studying "too small of a group." However, once I received the grant, I was forced to learn on my own how to navigate the Investigational Review Board (IRB) process. While this was an excellent learning experience, it was frustrating because I had to submit IRB applications to both our university and the Indian Health Service IRB offices. The two offices could not agree upon a common informed consent form. It took six months of negotiation between the two IRB offices to finally get this form approved! Eventually this early research activity paid dividends.

As I started exploring other research opportunities, it became clear that, as an economically disadvantaged state, New Mexico had several underserved populations. I decided that studying the use of pharmaceutical products and services among underserved populations would be a good research focus to have. As a matter of fact, this is my current research focus. Initially, there were several research projects that could be done, but I did not know which ones to choose and how to make research opportunities a reality. Ideas for projects presented themselves through college routing mail (what is this?), but during my first year on the job I was completely lost in terms of whom to approach for help with projects. For example, I had read that the use of herbal medicines was rampant in the New Mexican elderly. This prompted me to want to conduct a survey investigating the psychosocial predictors of the use of herbal medicines in this population. I did not pursue this project until a year ago, when I read a related study in a peer-reviewed journal written by a senior professor at our college who had an office down the hallway from mine. Here was someone with a similar research interest who had an office close to mine! If only I had known! In this environment, without a research mentor, I started taking on any project that looked interesting. As a result, I spread myself too thin.

I believe that it is very easy for junior faculty in pharmacy administration to get themselves into situations similar to mine, where they have too many research projects going on at one time. In the enthusiasm to help other pharmacy practice faculty who did not have research expertise but had wonderful practice-based research ideas, I took on too much. Graduate students who also needed research projects and training added to the list of projects. I was working very long hours because of the predicament in which I had put myself. At the beginning of this year, in addition to all my other teaching and administrative duties, I was involved in 19 research projects. There was no way I could terminate any of these! It was only then that I realized this kind of load was slowly infusing mediocrity into all my activities: research, teaching, service, and even my family life.

Part of the reason that I found myself in this situation was that I believed I needed to publish solely for tenure. I actually was told this repeatedly by senior faculty members. As a result, I agreed to get involved in any project that had even a remote possibility of yielding a peer-reviewed publication. Essentially, I thought, "The more publications, the better." Although I did not have a research focus at this point, this process did lead to a few publications. However, I believe that this is a trap that any junior faculty member can fall into at a research-intensive university. To guard against this, I would suggest carefully selecting research projects that have promise and are in an area of interest to the junior faculty member. If the projects are meritorious, publications will follow. The more of a research focus one has, the easier it becomes to garner research funds, simply because one has become recognized in that area of research. It is always good to remind ourselves that we publish to benefit the health care research community and/or patients rather than for the sake of tenure. Moreover, publishing for the sake of tenure will more likely lead to dissatisfaction and burnout than publishing for the enjoyment of scholarship.

As I mentioned earlier, since I didn't have a senior pharmacy administration faculty member to guide me, I had to elicit help from senior clinical pharmacy faculty members. A problem we had at our college was that there were very few senior clinical faculty members. I was fortunate that a very successful researcher, Dr. H. William Kelly, helped me considerably. His constructive criticism helped me realize that I had to focus my research efforts in order to be successful in the future. I am slowly starting to learn how to say "no" when asked if I want to participate in another research project.

One positive outcome of being overly zealous in accepting research opportunities was an invitation to be a research consultant for the New Mexico Medicaid Retrospective Drug Utilization Review (DUR) Program. From my perspective, consulting with the DUR Program has been beneficial since I have been able to keep my pharmacy as well as database research knowledge current. It is difficult to determine whether consulting would be beneficial to other junior pharmacy administration faculty members. I would suggest carefully considering the nature of the consulting position and the time commitment required. Consulting may not be a good option if it will stifle progress toward promotion at one's institution.

The slow process of completing my ongoing projects and carefully choosing future projects has only just begun. Along the road, I have had to seek out research mentors in other areas of pharmacy practice. It took me four years to figure out that I had spread myself too thin. Time will tell if I am successful in my research endeavors during the next few years.

TEACHING

The primary reason I joined academe was that I wanted to teach. Interactions with students both inside and outside class have always given me a sense of personal accomplishment. Of late, I have even injected a few of my research findings into my teaching in an attempt to find a bridge between the two.

My excessive teaching load when I first began my position at New Mexico was a consequence of numerous factors, not the least of which was the faculty attrition I mentioned earlier. Our school also has several curricula operating at the same time. I was responsible for a course in each program in my first semester. As a result, I was teaching in the B.S. pharmacy program, in the entry-level Pharm.D. program, in the track-through Pharm.D. program, and in the Ph.D. program in pharmacy administration.

My teaching methods have changed over the years. In my first year, I barely had enough time to prepare lectures. As some of our programs (B.S. and track-through Pharm.D.) were phased out, however, I was able to devote more time to devising innovative classroom strategies. I have tried several different types of in-class activities, such as cooperative learning, debates, and group presentations. In general, most of the in-class activities have worked well. There was only one occasion, when I conducted a debate about the pros and cons of a Pharm.D. degree in a B.S.-level course, that the debate got out of hand. I believe that this was because of the nature of the issue being debated and the fact that the class in which the debate was conducted was the last B.S. class in the college. In retrospect, it was not a very wise decision on my part.

In an attempt to take the active learning concept even further, I have had students get involved with projects outside of class. For instance, I have had students interview laypersons about pharmacy, conducted a pharmacy shadow program (where a student shadows a pharmacist for a day), and had students participate in various group projects. The group projects have been the most successful of these activities thus far. In these projects, students are required to maintain a reflective logbook about their activities and progress in the group project through the semester (1). Students have consistently indicated that the reflective logbook has helped them keep their projects on track as well as improve the quality of their projects. Another positive outcome that I have observed is that students within groups seem to have formed lasting friendships.

The only feedback that I have received to help me improve my teaching has been student evaluations. Students have been quite candid about what they have liked and disliked about my courses. Some of their comments have not been helpful. For example, some students have made comments about pharmacy administration courses being "pure psychobabble" and "a waste of a whole lot of credit hours." However, such comments only represent the views of a very small minority of students. Overall, my experience is that students are quite perceptive and are very capable of offering meaningful suggestions. I have incorporated some student suggestions, such as increasing the number of article evaluations in a research methods class. From my perspective, it has been heartening not to receive the same negative comment in two consecutive years. This probably indicates that it pays to heed student comments.

I stated above that only student comments have helped me improve my teaching. I am not saying that our department does not value teaching; it does. However, we do not have a formal peer teaching evaluation system in place. I have had senior faculty visit my class voluntarily, but I have never seen a formal evaluation of my teaching from any of them. Informally, senior faculty members have given me a few useful tips. I believe that every college should have a peer teaching evaluation and feedback system in place. Although research may be more important at some pharmacy schools, our mainstay is teaching students. Every pharmacy school will undoubtedly have a sentence in its mission statement indicating that it intends to provide quality education.

Mentoring new faculty in the area of teaching is important. Developing a course when one is just out of graduate school is a daunting task. There are so many issues to consider, like writing course and lecture objectives, researching the literature for lecture material, preparing succinct lecture notes and audiovisuals, effectively delivering lectures, and writing exam questions that reflect the objectives. Initially, I would suggest modeling lectures on those of former professors. Some of my former professors even allowed me to use their lecture notes. As time passes and lecture materials become obsolete, however, there is no substitute for reading the literature. Colleagues from other schools that one has met at professionals meetings can be a good source of teaching advice.

The issue of graduate education and teaching has been a strained one. The number of pharmacy administration faculty in our college has been based on the teaching load in the professional program. As our graduate program in pharmacy administration has grown, the department chair has come to realize that we need more faculty members to help with the teaching load in this program. Graduate student instruction was historically treated as a service-based activity. This has changed after several discussions with an understanding department chair. Graduate student instruction is now recognized as a teaching activity rather than a service-based activity. Polite persistence has paid off!

One aspect of teaching that I have thoroughly enjoyed is the student-centered problem-based learning (SCPBL) courses that we conduct every semester at our College of Pharmacy. These courses provide students with patient-based cases to "solve" with other group members. The instructor's duty is to act as a facilitator and tutor. These cases have given me an opportunity to revisit the information I learned and forgot in pharmacy school several years ago. Moreover, it has been wonderful to see students motivate themselves to learn while "solving" a patient case as a group.

In spite of my teaching load and my research schedule, I have been able to serve on several committees both within and outside our college. I outline in the next section my experiences with service-related activities.

SERVICE

In addition to research and teaching, I have been involved in a number of service-related activities. Faculty attrition has lead to my appointment on several faculty search committees, as well as college standing and ad hoc committees. My tenure on committees has been very useful in helping me to learn college and university policy and procedures. I believe that these committee appointments also helped me understand the views of other professors at our college.

The two most challenging committees on which I have served within our college have been the curriculum and graduate studies committees. Working on tasks for these committees has been extremely time consuming. For the Curriculum Committee, the process of phasing out our B.S. and track-through Pharm.D. programs and introducing the new entry-level Pharm.D. program has been especially tricky in terms of creating an environment in which the students in the programs being phased out were not neglected. With the new entry-level Pharm.D., we have had to make continual changes to both the didactic and experiential criteria for the program to run smoothly.

My role as the chair of the pharmacy administration graduate program has required me to serve on the Graduate Studies Committee. This was a difficult and frustrating role to fill, primarily because, at the time, we were struggling with recruiting and maintaining quality students. As a fresh Ph.D. graduate myself, at times I felt completely lost. However, serving in this capacity has been one of my most fruitful endeavors. By trying to emulate other established graduate programs in our geographic area, we have been able to raise our graduate student enrollment from 4 to 11 students in a span of 4 years. Additionally, we have been able to secure four college-funded graduate assistantships in the past four years.

At the Health Sciences Center level, I have served on the Clinical Process Improvement Committee (CPIC) for our university hospital. Serving on the CPIC has enabled me to get a flavor of how bureaucratic institutions operate. The most important outcome of serving on this committee has been the contacts it has allowed me to make with committee members outside the College of Pharmacy. Within the university I have also served as the advisor for the Indian Students Association. It has been inspiring to interact with many bright young Indian students who have been successful in obtaining good jobs.

Outside our university, I have served on national and state-level committees. The most positive outcome of serving on committees outside the university has been the opportunity to network with colleagues around the country. I believe networking with colleagues at other institutions has helped me share ideas and make professional contacts that may be helpful in the future. In my opinion, networking is an important activity that other junior faculty may wish to embrace.

Looking back over the last four years at the number of service-related activities that I have been involved in, I would have to agree with my department chair's last annual evaluation summary statement that said, "Simply, too much." I must confess that I have had difficulty refusing service-related committee assignments for fear of offending my more senior colleagues. On the other hand, I believe that these activities have allowed me to develop and maintain strong professional relationships with my colleagues that could potentially help me in the future. Hopefully, my service-based activities will become more streamlined and manageable in the future as I slowly learn the difficult art of saying "no" when asked to serve on a committee.

MENTORING

If not completely understood, mentoring can be a dirty word. Too often junior faculty at our college believe that a mentor is someone who will literally hold your hand, take you to the water, and make you drink. This is a fallacy. A mentor can only guide you, not do your work for you.

In my opinion, a mentor is someone who can help a junior faculty member navigate the complexities of beginning an academic position. The mentee, in turn, must pull his or her own weight. It is helpful if the mentor and mentee specialize in similar areas. Unfortunately, we did not have a senior faculty member in the pharmacy administration area during my first four years at the UNMCOP. This resulted in my seeking advice from several individuals on different aspects of my academic experience. So far, this approach seems to have been successful.

As I mentioned earlier, I sought the advice of a clinical pharmacy professor for my research. I have frequently asked for advice from a faculty member in the College of Medicine and from our department chair for my administrative (service) duties. I have even asked for advice from our dean from time to time. All of these individuals have been more than happy to help. Essentially, one may have to find multiple mentors for different purposes. An important point to note is that one has to search for mentors; they do not come to you on their own. This advice would be valuable at a school like ours, where a formal mentoring system did not exist when I joined the faculty. When a formal mentoring system exists, it may be possible for a senior faculty member to guide a junior faculty member to the right individuals, depending on the needs of the mentee.

In addition to my research, teaching, service, and mentoring experiences, there are other important issues that I have faced during the last four years in my faculty position. These are collegiality and university interface, the terror of tenure, and a supportive dean. I will briefly outline these in the next section.

OTHER IMPORTANT ISSUES

Collegiality and University Interface

I consider myself fortunate to have made so many professional contacts within the College of Pharmacy, within our Heath Sciences Center, and across the entire university campus. I believe that this indicates the willingness of professors in other disciplines to collaborate and to share ideas across the University of New Mexico campus. At the Health Sciences Center level, we have had Thanksgiving and Christmas lunches and musical performances for faculty in our medical mall. This has given me an opportunity to meet other faculty in a nonthreatening and relaxed atmosphere. Within the College of Pharmacy, the students and faculty have had frequent picnics. This has given faculty and students an opportunity to interact at a personal level. As one student once told me at one of these picnics, it allows students to get a chance to see that "faculty are human too!" I believe that it is important for colleges to conduct such social functions. It gives faculty and students an opportunity to feel a sense of belonging.

In spite of the many examples of collegiality I have described throughout this paper, relationships with other faculty are not without conflict. When it comes down to vying for fixed college resources, things can get ugly. For example, I was once told by a senior basic pharmaceutical sciences faculty member that "pharmacy administration and quality are an oxymoron." Worse still, the comment was made in the presence of students. Another faculty member informed me that there was nothing I could do about the situation because the senior faculty member was tenured and I was not. I must confess that this episode troubled me. However, I think these rare episodes can occur at any pharmacy school. I do not think this is in any way typical behavior of basic pharmaceutical sciences faculty. It is more a function of an individual's opinions. Several other basic sciences faculty members at our college have voluntarily made an effort to understand the issues that pharmacy administration addresses. Rather than dwell on this negative situation, I have used this experience to motivate me to perform better.

The Terror of Tenure

Tenure. The very word sends a shudder down most junior faculty members' spines. Many of my colleagues have mentioned to me that the tenure process is so vague that it is difficult to figure out what one really needs to do to get tenure. I have heard from others that some senior faculty members have used tenure as blackmail to get junior faculty to do things for them.

I have never felt threatened by the concept of tenure. I cannot say for sure how the Promotion and Tenure (P&T) Committee at our college makes its decisions, but I went through a pretenure review last year and passed. My opinion is that two faculty members cannot be compared (even if they are from the same department) when a tenure decision is made. The comparison is really between the achievements of the faculty member in question and a school's tenure criteria. To that effect, I followed the criteria that were given to me when I submitted the evaluation packet for my pretenure decision. Unlike other faculty members, who have indicated that the guidelines do not provide much direction, I found them quite helpful. The criteria were sometimes vague, but I think they were designed that way to allow the P&T Committee some flexibility in making decisions. I come up for tenure next year. Time will tell if my assessment of the tenure process was accurate or too naive!

A Supportive Dean

It would be remiss of me not to include a description of my professional relationship with the dean in an account of my experiences over the last four years. My dean has been very supportive of the activities of the pharmacy administration graduate program at our college. He or she has always made it a point to praise our work. As I mentioned earlier, I have even used him or her as a mentor when dealing with difficult administrative duties. Since my experiences have been unique, without a supportive dean not much of what I have been able to achieve as a junior faculty member would have been possible.

FINAL THOUGHTS

As I think of my trials and tribulations over the past four years, the positives outweigh the negatives. I am a better person and faculty member for the trials I have endured. The tribulations have reminded me that no job is a bed of roses. However, having overcome them has reminded me that my job has not been a bed packed with thorns. As my aspirations and goals change and mature, I may seek other faculty positions. The experiences I have had will help me shape my future.

I started out at the University of New Mexico not knowing exactly what would be expected of me in my research endeavors. Although I believe that I have been somewhat successful, I have become involved in too many research projects. Recently, a clinical faculty member has helped me understand how I can focus my research. My teaching activities, while almost unmanageable at first, have really kept me motivated. The interaction with students has been precious. My service-related activities have allowed me to make a number of very good professional contacts. Several mentors have been more than willing to help me, even when our college did not have a formal mentoring system in place.

When I think of all the wonderful relationships I have had with faculty and students, I am reminded of Dr. Joseph Wiederholt, the AACP Distinguished Faculty Member for 2000, who said, "Pharmacy educators are amongst the wealthiest people on Earth" in terms of the quality of their relationships. So, for those who feel their faculty positions stink, just like I did when I started out, think again: every cloud does have a silver lining.

REFERENCE

1. Gupchup GV, Mason HL, Foss M. The use of a reflective logbook to facilitate dynamic evaluation of activities in a group project. J Pharm Teach. 1995; 4(4):47-59.

Life and Times of a New Social and Administrative Sciences Faculty Member

Ana C. Quiñones

WHY ACADEME?

Choosing a career in academe was a "safe" and perhaps logical choice for me. My dad had been a Professor of Mathematics at the University of Puerto Rico, Mayaguez campus, for most of his life. My sister is an Associate Professor of Food Chemistry at the University of Puerto Rico, Utuado campus. I, however, am the only one in the family with a Ph.D. You could say that I went into an academic career having some idea of what to expect. Ultimately, I feel that academe provides a path where I could have the flexibility to achieve my major goals in life: having a job where I could help others and having a family. That's the reason I have selected this area as my professional path.

This was certainly not the way I envisioned my life to be ten years ago when I started graduate studies after pharmacy school. Back then, I remember resenting people's comments that pharmacy was a good career path for women: "After all, you can work part-time and still have a profession!" I think part of the reason I went to graduate school was to

---

Ana C. Quiñones, Ph.D., is Assistant Professor of Pharmacy Administration, Department of Pharmaceutical Sciences, School of Pharmacy, Massachusetts College of Pharmacy and Allied Health Sciences, 179 Longwood Avenue, Boston, MA 02115-5896 (E-mail: aquinones@mcp.edu).

[Haworth co-indexing entry note]: "Life and Times of a New Social and Administrative Sciences Faculty Member." Quiñones, Ana C. Co-published simultaneously in *Journal of Pharmacy Teaching* (Pharmaceutical Products Press, an imprint of The Haworth Press, Inc.) Vol. 9, No. 1, 2002, pp. 61-71; and: *Handbook for Pharmacy Educators: Getting Adjusted As a New Pharmacy Faculty Member* (ed: Shane P. Desselle and Dana P. Hammer) Pharmaceutical Products Press, an imprint of The Haworth Press, Inc., 2002, pp. 61-71. Single or multiple copies of this article are available for a fee from The Haworth Document Delivery Service [1-800-HAWORTH, 9:00 a.m. - 5:00 p.m. (EST). E-mail address: getinfo@haworthpressinc.com].

© 2002 by The Haworth Press, Inc. All rights reserved.

differentiate myself from most of my female classmates, who I felt had that "part-time" mentality. I considered myself more career-driven than most of my cohorts back home. Pharmacy would be more than an occupation for me. I did not go into pharmacy looking for a professional part-time job. However, four years ago, when I was told that my faculty position was going to be an academic (nine-month) appointment, I felt happy about securing a job that could allow me to have time to enjoy my future family and still be considered a full-time professional. I figured once I was married and had children, I could actually spend the summer months with them if I kept my nine-month appointment. How ironic! I have obtained all of this education and, at some level, I am still hoping to achieve what my college classmates got many years ago: a family of my own. Since I was hired, however, most of my colleagues have been given the option to switch to 12-month contracts, and most of them have done so. Today, I am actually one of the few nine-month faculty members left at the School of Pharmacy. I do spend considerable time during my summers performing school-related work for professional development and preparation for promotion. I am not going on the "mommy track" just yet, but if I ever get there, I will do it with no major regrets.

WHY MCPHS?

During the fall 2001 semester, I will have started my sixth year as an Assistant Professor of Pharmacy Administration at the Massachusetts College of Pharmacy and Health Sciences (MCPHS) in Boston, Massachusetts. I have an academic year, non-tenure-track appointment at this urban, private, teaching-intensive institution. The School of Pharmacy at MCPHS is divided into two departments: Pharmacy Practice and Pharmaceutical Sciences. I belong to the Pharmaceutical Sciences Department, which encompasses medicinal chemistry, pharmaceutics, pharmacology, and the social and administrative sciences (SAdS). This configuration is quite different from my graduate school, which was a public, research-intensive institution in Indiana where the SAdS was a part of the Pharmacy Practice Department. But these differences did not bother me. After all, part of the reason I came here is because I was looking for something different from what I had experienced before. I think the fact that I did graduate research in the area of pharmacists' career choices helped me select MCPHS. I was looking for an environment that would suit my favorite parts of an academic job, such as teaching, and would not be as demanding in other areas, such as research. Even my advisor in graduate school recognized that this might be a good choice for me.

I am one of five female faculty members in my department and the youngest of all members. The Department of Pharmacy Practice, on the other hand, has more females, younger faculty, and almost four times as many members. I can honestly say that faculty in my department have been very cordial and respectful. I know that some of them do not quite have a grasp of what the SAdS are all about, but they do understand that our discipline is research oriented, like theirs. That is the rationale for the departmental distribution in our school.

During my first departmental and schoolwide meetings, I would barely talk. I was more interested in hearing others talk, making mental impressions of their characters. I also wanted to determine "the right procedures" to follow and the behaviors that seemed to be conducive to positive interactions in my workplace. Now that I have figured out an effective communication style, I feel more willing to voice my opinion or make a contribution during group discussions. I would say it took me about a semester to learn the lines of communication at my institution, and my mentor was very helpful in this area. I feel that being cautious at the beginning was a wise choice. I found out that most people prefer honest, straightforward conversation, but there are always exceptions!

This is my first "real" job. MCPHS was one of two institutions with which I interviewed just before finishing my graduate studies. I recall being very nervous about my interview, but those who interviewed me were very gracious, understanding, and helpful. Having an SAdS background, I value the importance of interpersonal relations greatly. I felt and still feel that this is one of the greatest assets of the institution for which I work. Ever since my interview, I have had a really good feeling about MCPHS. I felt that I could fit into this academic environment. I believe the people I interviewed with had a lot to do with my decision to come to MCPHS. Once I accepted my position, my new group of colleagues (especially those within SAdS) made themselves available. They met me when I went apartment hunting with my mother and offered suggestions on where to live around Boston. Once I moved in, a colleague even helped me transport boxes from my apartment into my new office.

Over the years, the opportunity to develop both professional and social relations with a number of colleagues at MCPHS has helped me shape my academic persona. I interact quite often, on a casual basis, with some of the clinical and basic sciences faculty, as well as faculty members from other schools within the college. For example, a faculty member across the hallway from my office belongs to the nursing department. I have to admit that, besides the men in the SAdS group, I mostly interact on a social basis with female faculty of varied backgrounds. I find it harder to relate on a personal level to other male faculty members, even though some of them were hired at the same time I was hired and we are fairly close in age. Perhaps I look for many informal mentors of my own gender because I need the female point of view on academic life. What I value most from these interactions is the opportunity to listen to and be reminded of different points of view, as I live in a very diverse city and I interact with students of varied backgrounds on a daily basis. I consider my small group of colleagues who have allowed me to be part of their existence at MCPHS quite a blessing.

Most of my professional interactions happen within my own discipline or with colleagues with whom I share interests or courses. I would consider these interactions quite positive. For example, my involvement in a course cotaught with a faculty member from the Pharmacy Practice Department made possible a number of poster presentations and a publication. It also allowed me to look into potential areas of research I had not explored previously. Some of the most important professional relations are those with mentors, who are always looking after my professional development.

MENTORING

When I was hired, the head of my department decided to assign each of the new junior faculty in the pharmaceutical sciences to a formal mentor. Although I did not select my mentor, I am very satisfied with the assignment and probably would have chosen him. My mentor was the senior-most faculty member within the SAdS and the person in charge of the search committee when I interviewed for the job. We met at regular intervals to discuss my progress or just to chat. We shared similar educational experiences; we both had Ph.D.s from Midwestern schools of pharmacy with social/administrative sciences graduate programs, whereas most of our SAdS faculty at MCPHS had degrees from nonpharmacy schools. However, the differences–namely, his years of experience in academe–were what mattered. He helped me make a smooth transition from a large university setting into a small, independent school environment. He pointed out the pros and cons of the institution, as well as its lines of communication and power. I view my mentor as a wise brother who offers me advice but does not expect me to follow all of his suggestions word by word. To this day, I stop by his office to update him on my academic and personal life and to hear his valuable advice. Luckily, he always has the time to listen.

Three years after I was hired, it was decided that all junior faculty at MCPHS were to have a PAT (Peer Advisory Team) comprised of two senior faculty members. The main goal of the PAT is to provide formal mentoring to those junior faculty members previously without mentors (a concern for other departments at my institution). I kept my original mentor and added a female full professor from the School of Arts and Sciences as my second PAT member. I selected her because she is involved with the SAdS course I coordinate. Moreover, she was the first person I interviewed with when applying for my position, and I knew then that she was interested in my progress within the institution. I meet at least twice per semester with my PAT, as I have decided to go up for promotion in the fall of 2002. I enjoy the notion of having two mentors instead of one. One of the main advantages of this arrangement is having the wisdom of two professors with a proven track record at the institution. As a result of their qualifications, they both belong to many PATs within the school. I have no disadvantages to report on the PAT system. Since PATs guide junior faculty, one of their main objectives is to help faculty prepare for the promotion process. According to the school's faculty manual, junior faculty can go up for promotion after four years of employment, provided they meet the criteria for teaching, research, and service.

TEACHING, RESEARCH, AND SERVICE

MCPHS is a teaching-intensive institution; however, we are also expected to show progress in the areas of research and service to get promoted to the next level. Although the college does not give tenure, promotion guidelines are comparable to those of tenure-track schools. Moreover, after a successful probation period of four years, faculty can earn multiple-year appointments depending on their level. For example, I have received two-year appointments until I get promoted to the associate level. I think that the purpose of these multiple-year appointments is to provide a quasi-tenure contingent with one's promotion level within the institution. The factors of not having tenure and multiple-year contracts have not had any specific impact on my career-related attitudes thus far.

The faculty manual currently states that applicants can be up for promotion after four consecutive years of work at MCPHS. Applicants for promotion have to show outstanding contribution in two of the areas under consideration and significant contribution in the third one. The faculty manual contains no other specific criteria, perhaps because this document applies to all faculty members at the school, which includes arts and sciences, health sciences, and pharmacy. My recent meetings with my PAT indicate that I am doing well in the areas of teaching and service and that I should pay a little more attention to building on research.

In my first year of employment, I was exempt from service activities and was given a smaller teaching load in order to transition into my new role as a junior faculty member. I was expected to teach two sections of "Introduction to Health Care Delivery" (SAS 220), (one in the fall and one in the spring). I also was expected to develop an elective course in an area of interest or team teach the management course during the spring semester. I sat in the management course during the fall semester and quickly decided that teaching my own elective would be something that I would enjoy much more. I developed a special topics course, "Career Planning, Development and Management" (SAS 321), although it was not offered that spring due to an insufficient number of students registered. Instead, during the spring semester of my first year, I audited the elective course "A Survey of Alternative and Complementary Healing Practices" (PHA 390) and worked on a proposal for an in-house grant. Luckily, my department chairperson seemed supportive of my pursuing these various interests.

By my second year, I had a better idea of what my teaching responsibilities would be. I spent the following three years teaching all the aforementioned courses. After my first year, my involvement with these three courses increased, and currently I teach nine credits (or three course sections) per semester. Last year, I taught two sections of SAS 220 in the fall and one in the spring, I cotaught a section of PHA 390 in the fall and one in the spring, and I taught one section of SAS 321 in the spring semester. I am in charge of coordinating the various sections for SAS 220, which includes planning meetings for all instructors involved with the course (three or four on any given semester); we address the content and other specifics of the course to ensure homogeneity among sections.

I have discussed my teaching load with junior faculty in other schools of pharmacy, and I have been told that this is considered a heavy teaching load. This makes sense, since I am at a teaching-intensive institution. I do not mind the teaching load itself because I enjoyed the daily interactions with students a great deal. However, as the years at MCPHS progressed, I was expected to do more in the area of service and to maintain a certain level of scholarly activity. I believe that the ability to succeed at juggling these three aspects of an academic job is what helps one reach that level where one becomes "promotable." I realize that it is quite a challenge to keep the same level of achievement in all of these areas. So far, assessment of my teaching has not been hurt. Student evaluations of my teaching have been consistently positive and encouraging.

Nowadays, I find myself thinking of ways to increase my scholarship (a.k.a. research) while maintaining my current teaching and service levels. When I was first hired, I felt as if I had the time and energy to be involved in many scholarly pursuits. For example, I applied for and received an in-house "mini grant" to start developing a research area during my first year at MCPHS. The topic of my grant was a continuation of my doctoral dissertation. This grant allowed me to hire an undergraduate student to help with clerical work and paid a small stipend for the time I would spend on this project during the summer months. I did most of the data entry during the summer with the help of a second student who enrolled for undergraduate research credits. Although I was on academic appointment, I found myself going to work even during the summer, since this was the best time to devote to this project and I had a stipend paying for this time. The difference was the ability to set my schedule (and the students').

I enjoyed working with these students, but the experience made me wish we had a graduate program. After all, having graduate students keeps faculty involved in scholarly endeavors, even when these endeavors are not specifically theirs. I have tried to compensate for the lack of graduate students by allowing undergraduate students to do research with me. So far, I have had mixed results and have decided that, unless the student shows real commitment and interest for the experience, I am not going to accept every student who wants to do undergraduate research as an alternative to an elective course. When I made this decision, I felt that I was being selfish, but I also knew that I could spend a significant amount of time trying to be nice to students.

The mini grant supported the only piece of research that I have done. I guess I lost that energy from my first year rather fast! Oddly enough, I ended up getting a small article out of this piece of research before I put together an article based on my dissertation. (I do not suggest anyone follow this order.) Nowadays, I try to get my scholarship through other venues, and I jump at any opportunity that would entail a worthy entry on my curriculum vitae. As my date for potential promotion comes near, I am trying to put together materials for publication based on efforts other than survey research. Since my institution is not research intensive, I am hoping that these other scholarly endeavors are weighed as positively as survey research in the promotion review process. I have to admit that although I went through a rigorous pharmacy administration graduate program, I have never had the inclination to go into a "publish or perish" working environment. By "publish or perish" I am referring to producing publications that are based on research, as opposed to teaching. My only concern is making sure that my scholarly activities are adequate to ensure I get a promotion in 2002.

As far as service activities are concerned, you could say that my service involvement has really come to fruition during the last two years. Until then, I had only been involved with participation on smaller subcommittees and advising students. Advising is one of the main service duties for many faculty members at MCPHS. Starting my second year of employment, I was assigned about 20 student advisees. My responsibilities as an advisor entail ensuring that students are following an adequate course progression according to their plan of study. Advisors are supposed to sign the students' registration forms each semester. Moreover, advisors are sent copies of the students' final grades as well as their warning notes if they appear to be failing a course. When I was first told about my advising responsibilities, I was quite apprehensive. It felt like I had to be a cross between a mini registrar and a college counselor. I felt like I was not the best person to do this job; after all, I did not even know the pharmacy curriculum off the top of my head. I know that someone else must have felt the same way and made his or her voice heard. During my third year, we were offered advising workshops and given a user-friendly advising handbook. All of these were helpful, but at times my advisees would come with issues I could not deal with at all. I would turn to my mentor for advice on advising, and he was quite helpful. Nowadays, I feel a bit more comfortable about my advising duties. I do not advise students as well as some of my colleagues, but I feel like I am improving and getting the hang of it. I have even helped newer faculty members with their questions about the advising process.

My other significant areas of service involvement include: coadvisor of the Academy of Students of Pharmacy (ASP), member of the Curriculum Committee and delegate to the American Association of Colleges of Pharmacy (AACP). My responsibilities as advisor for ASP include attending its meetings and functions at the college and providing guidance in those areas where I can. In 2000, I accompanied the students to the ASP Midyear Regional Meeting for Region 1 in Albany, New York, and to the Annual Meeting in Washington, DC. Having a coadvisor is very helpful, as this colleague is more experienced with advising student groups and is well connected with the state association. Moreover, we can take turns at attending student events in case of scheduling conflicts. I thoroughly enjoy my involvement with ASP. Since I was a member when in pharmacy school and I have been to every APhA meeting since 1991, I feel being an ASP advisor is a logical extension of my involvement with APhA. I think the students appreciate the fact that my coadvisor and I are really getting involved with the group and not just using this title as another line on our curriculum vitae.

I found out about my appointment on the Curriculum Committee when I read my yearly contract two years ago. I asked my department chair about this appointment, as I had never been involved with a "major" committee within the college. I was told that it was time for me to get involved in major committees, as this type of involvement is looked upon favorably in the promotion process. That seemed reasonable. But when the fall semester started, I found out that they wanted me to be secretary of the committee! I had never served on this committee, and suddenly I was expected to furnish minutes based on what was being discussed during the meetings? I discussed this matter with one of my mentors and was advised to decline the secretary appointment. My mentor agreed that the committee work itself was a big responsibility and that my development within the committee would be best served if I did not become the secretary until the following year. So I said that I would not do it. This answer was not well received by the leaders of the committee, so I ended up doing what reasonable people do when they want to build positive working relationships: I compromised. I agreed to be secretary after my first semester on the committee. I took my appointment seriously and, as a result, have been complimented on my good work as secretary. However, after a year as the committee's secretary, I made it clear that it was time for someone else to take over this function. Most committee members agreed that one year as a secretary is reasonable, especially when the Curriculum Committee meets every other week year round, including summer.

I decided to run for alternate delegate for AACP while on a "promotion-driven spell." If I am going to get promoted, I need to make sure that I have enough service activities included in my vitae. Although I was already involved with advising, the Curriculum Committee and ASP, I figured that being involved with AACP would be a good move, especially since this is an appointment where I get to interact with delegates from other schools. I had been a member of AACP since graduate school, so I felt comfortable in undertaking such an assignment. One of my motivations for running for this position was to build a solid service section on my CV, but I also felt I could make a contribution in this area. I consulted with my mentor (who had been a delegate in the past), and he agreed this was a good choice for me. The school of pharmacy elects an alternate delegate for AACP every year. The alternate then becomes the delegate the following year.

REFLECTIONS ON MY ETHNICITY

I am one of only a few female Latino Ph.D.s in pharmacy academe. I have never felt much different from anyone else due to my gender or ethnicity while in graduate school or at my current job. I do not think that my unique demographic characteristics make me an expert on multicultural issues or entitle me to any preferential treatment. After all, I strongly believe that many of the issues I have described in this article are universal themes that all of us in academe face at some point in our careers.

One of the main cultural differences I have experienced during my ten years in the United States relates to attitudes toward life and work. I come from a culture where there is no "Protestant work ethic" or set of "workaholic" values. Living in the U.S., I have found myself striving to find a happy medium between these differing work-related attitudes. Some of these differences are very useful as examples in my elective career development course.

Being bilingual has provided me with the opportunity to get involved in unusual undertakings. For instance, last spring I was invited to talk about pharmacy on a local Spanish-speaking television show. Last summer, I was invited to accompany the MCPHS president on a trip to a pharmacy conference in Cuba. During this trip, I had the opportunity to do a podium presentation, in Spanish, on the feminization of pharmacy practice in the United States. I was more nervous about this presentation than I have been about many others. The reason was that I had undertaken my graduate studies in the U.S. and had done all of my scholarly work in English. Therefore, I had to spend more time than usual to ensure that my Spanish was "scholarly enough." I am eternally indebted to my sister, who read all of my notes before I went to Cuba. As a result of this trip, the college plans to start collaborations with other schools of pharmacy in Latin America, namely, those in Peru and Cuba. I have been named Special Assistant to the President for Latin American Initiatives, and this spring semester, I am coordinating the academic portion of an exchange program with two professors and four pharmacy students from Peru. Never did I imagine that I could be involved in starting such collaborations five years ago!

REFLECTIONS

So far, working in academe has been a great career choice. That is not to say that I have not had times when I wished I were doing something else. I think this is part of human nature. Academe has more flexible hours than many career paths, but some weeks are just as exhausting as the most demanding nonacademic jobs. In my case, I have come to realize that my 9-month contract sometimes turns into 10 or 11 months. Pursuing a career in academe is not as much about the money as it is about achieving intangible assets. I am willing to put in extra time for as long as I feel that my efforts are going to benefit someone. Sometimes I benefit, since I spend some of my summertime writing articles for future publication. Other times, my students benefit, as I use the weeks before the fall semester starts to update course materials. Finally, my colleagues benefit, as I am willing to meet even when not on contract to plan activities that help them achieve some of their goals.

Probably the biggest drawback of an academic life is that the salary earned does not seem to correlate well to the amount of years spent in graduate school. Becoming a college professor is definitely not about the money . . . unless you do consulting or move up the administrative ladder. I know that my students will make more money right after graduation than I do, and that is fine. The way I see it, I might earn less money, but I have more flexibility in scheduling my time.

I have learned a lot about academic life since I started my job six years ago. One of the most important lessons I have learned is to never promise to do something that you are not sure you can fit into your schedule, no matter how good it may look on your curriculum vitae. It is quite embarrassing to have to call someone and admit that you cannot keep your promise. I have learned to schedule fun time for myself. I try to take at least one non-work-related trip every year. Finally, I have learned that even in an area like academe, where so many aspects of your job can be constant for many years (e.g., courses taught), there can be enough variety (e.g., committee assignments, new students every semester) to keep you interested.

Succeeding in Academe–Self-Management and Passion

Lon N. Larson

INTRODUCTION

I am honored to be writing the "old timer's" perspective on beginning a career in academe. I find the academic life to be very fulfilling. I love learning and being a part of a community of learners. I delight in working with students, and I am awed to find myself in a position to touch their lives. I believe that, as an educator, I am part of a noble mission and that society benefits from my work. The academic life is not a life of leisure; if done right, it requires lots of hard work, but the rewards are tremendous (nonmonetary rewards, that is). My theme is simple: moving up the ranks as a professor requires self-management–more specifically, being "flexibly focused" and balancing personal and community goals–but deriving fulfillment from the work requires passion. Before developing these ideas, I want to explain who I am and why I wanted to write this essay.

As I write this, I am in my seventeenth year of teaching. Before my academic career, I worked eight years in community health planning and health insurance. My discipline is social and administrative pharmacy. I have taught at two disparate institutions: the University of Arizona and Drake University. Scholarship and graduate education were

---

Lon N. Larson, Ph.D., is Professor of Social and Administrative Pharmacy at Drake University College of Pharmacy and Health Sciences, 2507 University Avenue, Des Moines, IA 50311-4505 (E-mail: lon.larson@drake.edu).

[Haworth co-indexing entry note]: "Succeeding in Academe–Self-Management and Passion." Larson, Lon N. Co-published simultaneously in *Journal of Pharmacy Teaching* (Pharmaceutical Products Press, an imprint of The Haworth Press, Inc.) Vol. 9, No. 1, 2002, pp. 73-83; and: *Handbook for Pharmacy Educators: Getting Adjusted As a New Pharmacy Faculty Member* (ed: Shane P. Desselle and Dana P. Hammer) Pharmaceutical Products Press, an imprint of The Haworth Press, Inc., 2002, pp. 73-83. Single or multiple copies of this article are available for a fee from The Haworth Document Delivery Service [1-800-HAWORTH, 9:00 a.m. - 5:00 p.m. (EST). E-mail address: getinfo@haworthpressinc.com].

© 2002 by The Haworth Press, Inc. All rights reserved.

my highest priorities at Arizona, while professional education is my prime concern at Drake. I was promoted from Assistant to Associate Professor at Arizona and promoted to Professor at Drake. I earned tenure at both institutions. I have been lucky enough to win some awards. At Drake, I have been named the university's Mentor of the Year and the Pharmacy Teacher of the Year. However, I am not a superstar. I don't consider myself a "natural" at academic duties. Perhaps this is advantageous in this assignment. As my mother used to tell me when I was having trouble learning something, "Sometimes the person who has to work hard at mastering a subject or skill can explain it better than the person who acquires the skill easily and without much effort." (These may not have been her exact words, but they convey the sentiment.) I've worked hard to become a better member of the academy; hence, I hope I can provide insights about academic life that the reader finds helpful.

Why did I find this project so interesting? First, I was thrilled at the opportunity to help junior faculty get acclimated to the academy. I have thoroughly enjoyed life as a professor. I have found it challenging, rewarding, and just plain fun. For me, it has been a great career, and I think it can be the same for many others (but certainly not everyone). What a great gift I would be giving if, through this essay, I helped a junior professor find the fulfillment that I have found in the academy. Unlike scholarly publications, which convey information but do little to influence the reader's life, this project provided me with the unique opportunity to write a personal narrative. In this forum, I could perhaps provide the reader with useful information or needed encouragement. In essence, I could serve as a mentor, and potentially assist junior faculty, through my writing.

Second, I love the university and what it represents: a community of learners–faculty as well as students–seeking truth, openly debating ideas, exploring and learning about themselves and their world. However, as its critics are quick to point out, the university is not perfect. Academic freedom and tenure have been abused; arrogance is too common; and accountability is perhaps too rare. The university can be improved. As with all institutions, if the university hopes to realize its potential and fulfill its societal purpose, it must have good personnel–especially good faculty. If my words could attract, retain, or enhance the performance of even one bright young faculty member, I would have provided a great service to an institution I love and a mission I support.

Third, this essay provided an opportunity to write about work. I think meaningful work is one of life's great blessings. I also have many unanswered questions about work: What is the relationship between one's work and self-fulfillment? What role does work play in finding meaning in life? What does a person gain, if anything, from working hard (or is it merely a syndrome requiring therapy)? Why does one person find a particular job satisfying while another finds it boring? What does one need to do to make his or her work meaningful? Given the importance of work in our lives, I believe questions such as these are worthy of contemplation.

In sum, my goal in this project is to provide food for thought (I am hesitant to label it as advice) that junior professors may find useful in getting adjusted to academic life and that senior professors may perhaps find useful in renewal. In so doing, I hope to stimulate readers to think about why they are in academe, what they hope to give others, and what they hope to gain for themselves. Given the diversity of the audience–including many academic disciplines and differing university missions–my comments are quite general. The issues and problems I discuss are common to all faculty. I do not get into the mechanics of teaching, scholarship, and service, which I assume the new professor already knows (or is quickly learning). The content of the essay is organized according to my two major themes: self-management and passion. In the interests of full disclosure, I must confess that I preach better than I practice. Every pitfall I discuss, I have experienced (and will likely do again).

As a final introductory comment, I want to clarify success and how it is measured. Success in academic life can be measured in a couple of ways. First, it can be measured by the receipt of tenure and/or promotions to higher levels of professorship. This is an "other-oriented" view of success. Performance in teaching, scholarship, and service is reviewed and evaluated by others and judged by them to be worthy of promotion and/or tenure. In like fashion, others may be impressed by a colleague who is promoted or tenured. While this type of success is critical for a long-term academic career (since, for many faculty positions, continued employment requires tenure), it should not become the basis for self-evaluation. The second way of measuring success is internal. This is an exercise in self-reflection, focusing on the question: Am I continuously improving my abilities to perform activities that I find enjoyable and meaningful? The external and internal assessments of success may not be congruent. While social forces emphasize the former, I think each of us needs to assess his or her own success, independent of what others may think (at least, to the extent that this is humanly possible). I encourage junior professors to look beyond tenure; achieving tenure or promotion is not the ultimate definition of success.

SELF-MANAGEMENT IN ACADEMIC LIFE

The function of management can be viewed as using resources to reach a goal. For the professor, the resources are time and energy, and the goal is "academic net worth." I use this phrase to refer to documented outcomes or accomplishments. A professor's academic net worth is detailed in his or her curriculum vitae and teaching portfolio and includes grants and publications, service activities, and teaching experiences and effectiveness. These documents are used in making promotion/tenure decisions. They also are what colleges review in selecting new faculty. Ultimately, it is academic net worth that is relevant in promotion and tenure reviews.

I include teaching portfolio because without it, I fear teaching receives too little attention, both in external assessments and in our own self-assessments. For scholarship, we have two widely understood indicators of performance: grants and peer-reviewed publications. These are detailed in the vitae. Similar indicators for teaching and service are not available; data in the vita are often limited to quantity of work in these areas, with no hint of quality or effectiveness. Thus, there is little incentive to improve teaching. For those who are primarily teachers (I am one), there is little chance to show the results of their efforts. A teaching portfolio rectifies this situation. It includes such information as teaching philosophy, teaching methods and their rationale, course syllabi, and data documenting teaching effectiveness. The portfolio allows teaching to play a larger role in academic net worth.

Professors, compared to other employees, are quite independent (but not totally independent, as discussed later). This independence is both good and bad. Independence is one of the most attractive features of being a professor. Professors can say what they want, choose the questions they want to explore and investigate, participate in their choice of service activities, and, within bounds, select the content they teach and the methods by which they teach it. The professor does not "punch a clock" or "take orders from a boss." Although the department chair may help set priorities and monitor progress, on a day-to-day basis, the professor is allowed to decide how to spend his or her time and mental energy.

Along with the independence, the professor has a very open-ended position description. The professor is responsible for teaching, scholarship, and service. While the priority assigned to each of these functions varies, every professor is doing some combination of these three functions. The problem is that each of these three has an insatiable appetite–each can consume all of a professor's time and energy. Every activity the professor performs can be enlarged or enhanced: a class session can be better planned, a manuscript or grant application can be revised and rewritten, comments on students' papers can be more detailed, more attention can be given to advisees, and the list goes on and on. These are all worthwhile activities (some affect the welfare of students and colleagues), and they deserve to be performed conscientiously. Given such an open-ended job description and the high level of independence in setting priorities, every professor faces the quandary of having too many things to do and too little time to do them.

I see two major dilemmas in self-management for the professor. One is to stay focused, but flexibly so. This apparent contradiction will be explained later. As the professor scurries about, trying to cope with a never-ending list of things to do (all of which can be improved), it's easy to become wrapped up in all the activity and lose sight of the desired objective. The situation may be likened to that of a bird flying south for the winter: what matters to the bird is how far it flies, not how many times it flaps its wings.[1] With all that they have to do and all the demands placed upon them, it's easy for professors to start "flapping around" and forget what they want to accomplish.

To help the professor stay focused, I think planning and self-monitoring are essential. This builds upon, and goes beyond, the annual faculty plans that many universities require. The goal here is not so much a neat-looking document as it is a usable road map. Every professor should have a work plan that specifies the activities that will be done and when. This work plan should be quite specific and detailed; the greater the specificity, the greater the value. In developing the work plan, the professor should thoughtfully answer these questions pertaining to output, effort, and personal development, respectively:

- What do I want to accomplish? What additions or changes will be made in my curriculum vitae or teaching portfolio?
- What activities will I perform and when? How will I spend my time?
- What skills do I want to improve?

A work plan is worthless if it is not accompanied by monitoring. Monitoring–comparing actual progress against what was anticipated–is essential if the professor is to focus on "the distance traveled." Regardless of how often formal reviews are done with the department chair, professors should frequently conduct self-monitoring, in which they critically assess their progress and prospects. These self-evaluations should be honest. In areas of deficiency, developing strategies to get back on track is more useful than merely justifying the lack of production. Ultimately, professors are judged on the basis of their output, their academic net worth.

A related issue is balancing focus and flexibility. Every professor is presented with unforeseen opportunities. These may be in teaching, but more likely, in scholarship or service. They may be very attractive, but as luck has it, they seldom fit precisely with the professor's plans. The professor is left with the dilemma: follow the plan (first choice) with its uncertainty (it may not work out as anticipated) or seize the new opportunity (second choice) that is certain. I think these are some of the most difficult decisions a professor makes, especially junior faculty. Deciding whether to pursue the opportunity requires thoughtful consideration of its cost and benefits. In assessing the benefits of an unforeseen opportunity, these questions may be helpful:

- Is it in an area of interest that I want to develop?
- How may it enhance my skills or reputation?
- Will it lead to other projects?
- Can the experience be used in some other fashion? For instance, a service activity may have publication potential, or contract research with little chance of publication may provide support for a graduate student.
- Will the project be enjoyable?

However, a new project comes with a cost, and an informed decision requires that this cost be considered. For the professor, the cost is the other opportunities that will be left undone because time is spent on the new endeavor; opportunity cost refers to opportunities lost. In other words:

- What project(s) will be delayed, discarded, or done less thoroughly if this one is pursued?

An example may help bring some of this to life. When I was asked to write this essay, I already had a full schedule. For the reasons detailed earlier, I found the project interesting. In addition, as a publication, it represented academic net worth. Yet, something would have to be sacrificed–a trade-off would have to be made. I don't know exactly what was left undone because of this essay, but the most likely suspects are a teaching innovation that I had planned to develop and fewer evenings at home with nothing to do. In essence, the cost of this essay was potentially less student learning, a weaker teaching portfolio, less time with family, and less sleep. A professor's most valuable assets are time and energy. They must be spent consciously and judiciously.

A second dilemma in self-management is the balance between individualism and communitarianism, in other words, the balance between "doing my own thing" and "being a team player." Faculty independence and academic freedom have their limits. Professors have responsibilities to their learning communities that go beyond enhancing their own academic reputation or net worth. Narrowly, this community responsibility can be seen as serving on university committees, but more broadly (and I believe more accurately), the responsibility involves improving the quality of learning that takes place within the university.

Trends in pharmacy education suggest a move toward communitarianism and broader community responsibilities for the professor, especially in teaching and program assessment. Many colleges have initiatives to improve learning, and as a result, professors may have to compromise their preferred teaching strategies for the betterment of the community. For instance, some schools offer integrated, interdisciplinary courses that require team members to collaborate–and compromise–on course design and teaching methods. Another initiative is making classes more active and shifting the perspective of classroom performance from teaching centered to learning centered. As a final example, if writing or speaking is emphasized throughout the curriculum, then many faculty from several disciplines are affected. The increased attention on assessing curricular outcomes also promotes communitarianism. Here, the curriculum is seen as a single entity rather than the sum of several independent components. As such, the assessment is of the collective efforts of the faculty. It encourages professors to work together, to see how their respective pieces of the puzzle can better fit together for the benefit of student learning.

The dilemma for the professor is to balance these community goals with the personal goal of acquiring academic net worth (documented outcomes). For example, grading and critiquing student papers may be essential for enhancing student learning but may generate little net worth. While time spent on this activity may benefit students and the community by improving the quality of learning, it does little to benefit the stature of the professor. Devoting time and energy to the learning community has an opportunity cost, which may be reduced personal credentials or less academic net worth. This poses a dilemma for colleges as well. If colleges expect professors to be committed communitarians and to spend more time on teaching and assessment–per the wishes of the community–then less time is available to generate academic net worth. Expectations concerning faculty performance for tenure or promotion may need to be adjusted. This is a very complex issue for individuals and institutions. I think it is worthy of personal reflection and public discussion.

I want to close this section on self-management with two bits of advice. One is highlighted by Franklin Roosevelt's rule that "energy is more efficient than efficiency" (1). In other words, at the core of being productive is hard work. Self-management without hard work is worth little. Self-management can augment hard work, but not replace it. The second point comes from advice I first heard in the context of baseball. It goes like this: "Sometimes you get in a slump, and nothing seems to go right. Other times, you get 'hot' and everything goes your way. You have to learn not to get too down on yourself during the slumps . . . nor too proud of yourself during the hot streaks."[2] I suspect every professor has both "slumps" (disinterested students, a manuscript or grant rejected) and "hot streaks" (great class discussion, teacher of the year, request to write a manuscript). Avoiding self-flagellation and self-aggrandizement improves the quality of academic work life.

PASSION IN ACADEMIC LIFE

The previous section described the importance of self-management in academic life and presented some thoughts on how to manage that life more effectively. While self-management may enable the professor to earn tenure and promotion, I am quite sure that self-management is not what makes an academic career meaningful. Rather, the meaning and joy of academic life derive from the attitudes of the professor–the passion and caring that he or she brings to the job. I believe three passions are important in finding fulfillment in an academic life (and perhaps all careers). These passions can apply to teaching, scholarship, and service, although my discussion focuses on teaching.

Fulfillment in academic life is enhanced if the professor has a passion for lifelong learning and continuous self-improvement. This may be phrased as striving for excellence. This passion brings freshness to work. No one wants to be in a rut or routine that, through its regularity and familiarity, grinds the joy out of work. Most of us will not experience the same kind of adventures as Professor Indiana Jones (nor may all of us want to), but even ordinary professorial work can be exciting and new. Scholarship, by definition, is exploring and testing new ideas. Teaching can be an exercise in lifelong learning and continuous improvement. For instance, using current theory and published research, teaching innovations are designed and implemented. Then their effectiveness is assessed, and revisions are made. This is scholarly teaching (2). (This is not the same as scholarship of teaching, which requires more external review.) When one considers the many elements involved in a course or other learning experience–assignments and student projects, classroom activities, assessing student performance, and evaluating teaching effectiveness–the learning potential of teaching becomes clear. I try to be a scholarly teacher, and I can vouch that it keeps teaching new and fresh. I learn every time I teach a course. As with most learning, not all the lessons are pleasant, but the process is never dull.

Second, fulfillment in academic life is enhanced with a passion for the welfare of students, that is, if the professor cares about his/her students. This passion has two aspects. One, the professor realizes the great influence that he or she can potentially have on students. In Robert Smith's words, it is the potential to "unleash the greatness" in a student (3). I, for one, am humbled by the magnitude of this power. Most of us can relate to this phenomenon more easily by considering the teachers who most influenced us, rather than by thinking of ourselves as the ones who can unleash greatness. The second aspect is that student-teacher relationships are welcomed and fostered by the professor (4). Students are novice learners and novice professionals; they need mentors and role models. Mentoring relationships–in which the teacher serves as a trusted guide or advisor for the student–can be very meaningful for both student and professor. Probably my fondest memories in academe involve working with or advising a student one-to-one. Mentoring relationships are perhaps easier and more commonly developed with graduate students, but they are equally meaningful when developed with undergraduate or professional students.

Third, fulfillment in academic life is enhanced if the professor has a passion for the value of education. How do individuals and society benefit from college education, and more specifically, pharmacy education? If a professor does not see the value of education, it's hard to imagine much fulfillment being derived from doing the work of a professor. Hopefully, professors see the value of what they teach and how it fits into the education of the student. For instance, I believe that pharmacy students benefit from a good, solid grounding in the social and administrative sciences because it enhances their abilities to be caring clinicians, advocates for the community's health, rational users of limited resources, and effective participants in shaping organizational and public policies. On a broader level, there is the value of the entire educational experience. The value of pharmacy education may be seen as extending beyond enabling the student to practice pharmacy competently, to providing the student with a liberal education that influences all aspects of life (3, 4). With such an education, students are better able to analyze and perhaps influence the events of their time and to reflect upon and savor the experiences of their lives. One professor cannot do this alone; but by working with others in the learning community, the individual professor can influence the entire educational experience of the student.

The professor's passion for teaching can be easily drained. This may be what afflicts older professors who seem to have lost their enthusiasm or zeal. (This is an affliction that concerns me greatly, since I am at or near the age of highest risk.) I mention two factors that I find draining. One is the inability to measure my effectiveness in teaching. We all need to see the fruits of our labors. We need that kind of feedback to keep working hard. I find the fruits of my teaching labors difficult to measure. I cannot easily assess the effects of my efforts on student learning, nor can I easily measure my progress as a teacher. I know I am working harder than ever, but I have little evidence of its effects. This makes it difficult to continue. A second drain is the disinterested student. Just as the enthusiastic student gives me energy, the disinterested one absorbs it. My energy level throughout a day is affected noticeably by the quality of classroom discussion. A good discussion gives me energy, while I am exhausted after a poor one. I wish I could grow a thicker skin without becoming callused. I think all professors need to accept the fact that they are not going to please all the students all the time.

In sum, if a professor has a passion for self-improvement, cares about the welfare of students, and believes in the value of education, he or she is likely to find fulfillment in academic work. As a professor, I see myself in the front lines of the fight against ignorance and closed-mindedness. I can imagine few causes as noble, and I can imagine no way to have a more fulfilling work life.

CLOSING COMMENTS

In closing, I think being a professor is just about the best job there is. As a means of summarizing my thoughts in the essay, here is the advice I have for the prospective or beginning professor:

1. Work hard. As my mother used to say, "You get out of it what you put into it." This is certainly the case in academic work.
2. Your resources are your time and energy. Use them wisely.
3a. Stay focused. Have a work plan and monitor yourself often.
3b. Be flexible. Seize opportunities when they arise, but remember that saying "yes" comes with an opportunity cost.
4. Think in terms of academic net worth (documented outcomes) in your curriculum vitae and teaching portfolio. This is the currency in which your value in academe is measured.
5. Contribute to your learning community (university and college). Improve the quality of learning that occurs there.
6. Balance #4 and #5. They are both essential, but not necessarily compatible.
7. Your influence as a teacher can be profound, so work hard at it.
8. Remember your purpose. It's much like bricklayers: one may focus on bricks and mud while another imagines the cathedral that is being built. The second finds more fulfillment.
9. Be passionate about what you do. Enjoy it. Have fun.

NOTES

1. The bird analogy was adapted from Edward Suchman, *Evaluative Research*.
2. Author unknown.

REFERENCES

1. Goodwin DK. No ordinary time–Franklin and Eleanor Roosevelt: The home front in World War II. New York: Simon and Schuster; 1994.
2. Hutchings P, Shulman LS. The scholarship of teaching: New elaborations, new developments. Change. 1999; (Sept/Oct):11-15.
3. Smith RE. Unleash the greatness. Am J Pharm Educ 1999; 63:436-41.
4. Smith RE. A free lunch pays for itself: The value of relationships in education. Address of the President, AACP, 2000.

Index

AACP. *See* American Association of Colleges of Pharmacy (AACP)
Academic freedom, 9-17
Academic support structures, 15-16
Academy of Students of Pharmacy (ASP), 68-71
ACCP. *See* American College of Clinical Pharmacy (ACCP)
American Association of Colleges of Pharmacy (AACP)
  Annual Meetings, 23-24
  Curriculum Committee, 68-71
  Grant Writing Program, 29
  Mentoring Program, 11-14
American College of Clinical Pharmacy (ACCP)
  Ambulatory Care Practice and Research Network (PRN), 28
  Grant Writing Program, 29
ASP. *See* Academy of Students of Pharmacy (ASP)
Associations, professional. *See* Professional associations
Autonomy, 32-33

Baker, P., 17
Barry, K., 17
Barzun, J., 47
BCPS. *See* Board Certified Phamacotherapy Specialists (BCPS)
Beamon, R., 39
Bellas, M. L., 17

Biglan, A., 6
Billings, D. A., 6
Board Certified Phamacotherapy Specialists (BCPS), 29
Boice, R., 6-7
Boyer, E., 47
Braxton, J. M., 6
Bultemeier, N., 19-33

Carnegie Research I Universities, 49
Certified Diabetes Educator (CDE), 28
Clerkship sites, 27-33
Cole, J., 17
Collegiality and university interfaces, 56-57
Continuing education, 29-33
Crawford, L. A., 17
Creamer, L., 17

Departmental structures
  mentoring activities and, 9-17
  of small departments, 49-54
Desselle, S. P., 1-7
Drake University, College of Pharmacy and Health Sciences, 73-83
Duquesne University, Mylan School of Pharmacy, 1-7
Dwyer, M. M., 6

Eddy, R. M., 17
Equilibrium, pretenure, 9-17
Ethnicity issues, 70-71

© 2002 by The Haworth Press, Inc. All rights reserved.

Faculty/staff retreats, 42-43
Feldman, D. C., 17
Flynn, A. A., 6
Foss, M., 59

Gaither, C. A., 6
Garaza, H., 6
Goal-setting, 19-20
Goodwin, D. K., 83
Grant writing, 29-33,43-45
Grillo, J. A., 6
Gupchup, G. V., 47-59

Hammer, D. P., 1-7
Hargens, L. L., 6
Health-related quality of life (HRQOL) questionnaire, 49
Hutchings, P., 83

IHS (Indian Health Service) Hospital, 49
Inmann, P. S., 6

Johnsrud, L. K., 6
Journals, keeping of, 19-20

Kelly, W. H., 51

Larson, L. N., 73-83
Latif, D. A., 6
Lemke, T., 17

Mason, H. L., 59
Massachusetts College of Pharmacy and Allied Health Sciences (MCPHS), 61-71
Menges, R. J., 6
Mentoring activities
    departmental structure and, 9-17
    formal vs. informal, 31-33
    at Massachusetts College of Pharmacy and Health Sciences (MCPHS), 64-65
    at Oregon State University, College of Pharmacy, 31-33
    peer mentoring, 40-41
    research vs. teaching, 12-16,49-54
    at Shenandoah University, 40-41
    in small departments, 49-54
    at University of Mississippi, School of Pharmacy, 11-16
Mission statements, 22

Nair, K. V., 6
National Institutes of Health (NIH), 3
Near, J. P., 6
New Mexico Medicaid Retrospective Drug Utilization Review (DUR) Program, 47-59
NIH. *See* National Institutes of Health (NIH)
Nonmonetary rewards, 73
Novo Nordisk Pharmaceuticals, Inc., 35

OHSU. *See* Oregon Health Sciences University (OHSU)
Olsen, D., 6,17
O'Neil, R. M., 17
Oregon Health Sciences University (OHSU), 22-33
Oregon State University, College of Pharmacy, 19-33
Orientation activities, 32-33
Outpatient clinics, 27

Passion, Rapport, Organization, Fairness (PROF) principles, 15-16
Patitu, C. L., 6

Index

PCAT scores, 44
Pharm.D. candidates
   research collaboration and, 44-45
   residencies and, 19-33
Pharmacy practice residencies, 19-33
Pharmacy schools
   Drake University, College of Pharmacy and Health Sciences, 73-83
   Duquesne University, Mylan School of Pharmacy, 1-7
   Massachusetts College of Pharmacy and Allied Health Sciences (MCPHS), 61-71
   Oregon Health Sciences University (OHSU), 22-33
   Oregon State University, College of Pharmacy, 19-33
   Shenandoah University, 35-45
   University of Arizona, 73-74
   University of Mississippi, School of Pharmacy, 9-17
   University of New Mexico, College of Pharmacy, 47-59
   University of Washington, School of Pharmacy, 1-7
Porter, D. W., 17
Portfolio creation and construction, 14-16
Practice vs. teaching responsibilities, 19-33
Pretenure equilibrium, 9-17
Primary care residencies, 19-33
PROF principles. *See* Passion, Rapport, Organization, Fairness (PROF) principles
Professional associations
   Academy of Students of Pharmacy (ASP), 68-71
   American Association of Colleges of Pharmacy (AACP)
      Annual Meetings, 23-24
      Curriculum Committee, 68-71
      Grant Writing Program, 29
      Mentoring Program, 11-14
   American College of Clinical Pharmacy (ACCP)
      Ambulatory Care Practice and Research Network (PRN), 28
      Grant Writing Program, 29
Professional credentials, 28-33

Questionnaires, Health-related quality of life (HRQOL), 49
Quiñones, A. C., 61-71

Rau, W., 17
Research activities and issues
   collaborative research, 20,45
   at Massachusetts College of Pharmacy and Health Sciences (MCPHS), 65-70
   mentoring activities and. *See* Mentoring activities
   pilot studies, 20
   small departments and, 49-51
   tenure and. *See* Tenure system and process
   vs. teaching activities, 12-16
Residencies
   pharmacy practice, 19-33,42-45
   primary care, 19-33
   research activities and, 43-45
   teaching and, 35-45
Retreats, faculty/staff, 42-43
Rimoldi, J. M., 9-17
Roosevelt, F. D., 80
Run-in periods, 20-33

Sandler, B. R., 6
Schools of pharmacy. *See* Pharmacy schools
SCPBL. *See* Student-centered problem-based learning (SCPBL)
Self-evaluation, 14
Self-management

career passion and, 80-82
description of, 73-75
fulfillment and passion in academic life, 80-82
functions of, 76-80
importance of, 82-83
introduction to, 73-74
Senior faculty perspectives, 73-83
Service activities, 65-70
Service issues, 15-16,30,41-42,54-55
Shenandoah University, 35-45
Shulman, L. S., 83
Small departments
  administrative support and, 58
  collegiality and university interface and, 56-57
  future perspectives of, 58-59
  introduction to, 47-49
  mentoring issues and, 55-56
  research issues and, 49-51
  service issues and, 54-55
  teaching issues and, 51-54
  tenure issues and, 57-58
Smith, R., 81
Smith, R. E., 83
Social support networks, 11-12
Sorcinelli, M. D., 6-7
Steers, R. M., 17
Stolte, S. K., 35-45
Student-centered problem-based learning (SCPBL), 54
Suchman, E., 83

Tack, M. W., 6
Teaching responsibilities
  grading and, 30-40
  lecture preparation, 36-39
  small departments and, 51-54
  at small universities, 35-45
  teaching philosophies and, 39-40
  vs. practice responsibilities, 19-33
Tenure system and process

academic process and, 9-17
academic support structures and, 15-16
contracts and, 20-22
departmental structure and, 9-17,20-22
goal-setting and, 19-20
mentoring activities and. *See* Mentoring activities
mission statements and, 22
at Oregon State University, College of Pharmacy, 19-33
Passion, Rapport, Organization, Fairness (PROF) principles, 15-16
portfolio creation and construction and, 14-16
pretenure equilibrium and, 9-17
research vs. teaching and, 12-16
run-in periods and, 20-33
self-evaluation and, 14
service components of, 15-16,30,41-42
in small departments, 57-58
surveys about, 9-10
teaching responsibilities and, 22-25
at University of Mississippi, School of Pharmacy, 9-17
  mentoring activities and, 11-16
vs. non-tenure track, 42-45

University of Arizona, 73-74
University of Mississippi, School of Pharmacy, 9-17
University of New Mexico, College of Pharmacy, 47-59
University of Washington, School of Pharmacy, 1-7

Wolfgang, A. P., 6
Wolverton, M., 14,17